Dr. Sebi Bible

The Complete Step-By-Step Guide to Cleanse, Detoxify Your Body, and Live an Ailments-Free Life Thanks to the Power of Herbal Remedies and Alkaline Diet

by

Lisa G Torres

Table of Contents

BOOK 1

Dr. Sebi Herbal

Dispensatory

The Alkaline Diet's main premise is that anything we eat has a neutral ph, a certain acidity, that may impact the pH level of your body. Your body's capacity to fight illness is influenced by your pH level, which has a significant impact on your physical wellbeing. The pH scale is simple to understand. It lies on a spectrum from 0 to 14, with 0 being the most highly acidity, 7 being neutral, and 14 being the most basic. The reverse of acid is the basic end of the spectrum, which is sometimes known as alkaline. A healthy body has a pH of 7.4, which is somewhat on the alkaline end of the pH scale. The human body produces waste products of metabolism on a regular basis. The Alkaline Diet's main goal is to make this debris as alkaline as feasible so that the system isn't pushed to cope with acidic material. The Alkaline Diet is basically a blood pH control diet.

When the body's fluids, especially the bloodstream, have too much acid, acidosis develops. When your tissues, particularly your kidneys and lungs, are unable to sustain your blood's optimal pH, an equilibrium that is an essential aspect of normal homeostasis, this process occurs. Acidosis may occur when the kidneys or lungs are damaged or diseased, impairing their capacity to keep a healthy, mildly alkaline pH. Acid accumulates in the system when the organs aren't working properly, as a consequence of the systems that helps in digestion, turn it into energy, and oxygenate your tissues.

Respiratory acidosis affects the lungs, as you would expect. Whenever we inhale and exhale, our lungs normally eliminate carbon dioxide from our system; however, if this mechanism is disrupted, surplus carbon dioxide accumulates in the body. Overweight and alcoholism both have an influence on pulmonary function and may lead to respiratory acidification.

The kidneys, on the other end, are involved in metabolic acidosis. Diabetes and obesity may make it difficult for the kidneys to remove surplus acid from the system, enabling it to build up in the bloodstream. The kidney's capacity to handle acidic waste products of metabolism is also affected by dehydration. This is also why the Alkaline Diet emphasizes drinking

plenty of fluids per day and abstaining from alcohol, which promotes the accumulation of acid in the blood. Acidosis may cause bone degeneration, kidney disease, and other renal issues over time.

Holistic medicine refers specifically to any medical practice that takes into account the whole person instead of one component. A holistic therapy, for example, considers the wellness of the brain, feelings, and soul in addition to the physical body. Dr. Sebi's naturalism and herbalism were closely associated with holistic medicine. Herbalism is at the crossroads of conventional and holistic medicinal practices. It investigates the inherent features of once-living plants and how they might be used to cause medically significant changes in the body. In the same manner that inorganic components create remedies in traditional drugs, herbalism strives for milder, cleaner ways to address health issues. This framework eliminates many of the negative consequences of adding synthetic substances into the body's living cells.

Herbal medicine precedes what we would now refer to as medicine. Herbalism was the forerunner of what would ultimately develop into modern medical science in olden history. Herbalism focuses completely on the varied therapeutic powers of herbs given as a cure, but many pharmaceutical organizations still employ herbs and plant compounds. Dr. Sebi's herbal teachings were centered on the African culture, with which he had a relationship thanks to his grandparents. Dr. Sebi created his supplement brand with the intention of converting plants into a much more conventional form that might contend more successfully with established medications, such as tablet form. His purpose, as well as the purpose of his Alkaline Diet, was to tackle these underlying problems at the cellular level.

In this book, we'll talk about how Dr. Sebi used alkaline medicinal herbs and plants to bring back the body's natural pH balance to heal common illnesses, including digestive problems, kidney, liver and pancreatic issues. We'll dive into a plethora of r. Sebi's recommended natural herbs to detox the major organs of the body and boost your immune system to gain health and wellness, how to use them, their origins and much more.

The Basics of Dr. Sebi's Alkaline Diet and Herbs

The Alkaline Diet didn't just appear out of nowhere. Dr. Sebi required a long time to completely establish his theory and therapy. Dr. Sebi understood there were reasonable alternatives to Medical practices from his early days when he looked to his Black culture and his grandma's herbal remedies for solutions. Dr. Sebi understood that he needed to discover a means to completely detox the body off of toxic elements by restoring the body's normal alkalinity. In memory of its creator, the regimen that Dr. Sebi alluded to as the "African Bio-Mineral Balance Diet" has subsequently been known as Dr. Sebi's Alkaline Diet. The Cell Foods site, which is approved by Dr. Sebi's business to offer his goods, describes their concept simply; as illnesses can only thrive in an acidic medium in the system, treating them with acidity, artificial medicines makes literally no sense.

Dr. Sebi was dedicated to cleansing and replenishing the body at the molecular level, allowing the body's natural defense processes to take over the repair and regeneration processes. Dr. Sebi believed that health begins at the molecular level, from within. The Alkaline Diet permits the body's natural healing mechanisms to function at their best by concentrating on organ detoxification. Dr. Sebi's herbal treatment replenishes deficient nutrients and revitalizes damaged tissues that have been destroyed by the degenerative, acidic condition. Impairment of vital organs implicated in the elimination of waste substances may result in diseases and have long-term consequences for one's health and wellbeing.

In this chapter, we'll look at Dr. Sebi's die philosophy, what we mean by herbs, their specific uses in cooking and for healing, etc., and what are their important parts that can be used therapeutically. We'll also highlight some important precautions you need to take before diving into Dr. Sebi's recommended medical plants and herbs for healing health issues.

Alfredo Bowman was the brains behind the Dr. Sebi Diet. He was a self-described healer and healer from Honduras who utilized food to enhance his wellbeing. Despite the fact that he is no longer alive, he nevertheless maintains a large following in the twenty-first century. He claims to have cured a variety of ailments utilizing plants and a stringent vegan diet as a result of his holistic approach. Before relocating to New York City, he established a treatment facility in his own country, where he had maintained his profession and expanded his clientele to include Michael Jackson, John Travolta, Eddie Murphy, and Steven Seagal, to mention very few.

His diet is similar to being vegan, although it is a highly rigorous version of it. There are many parallels to the standard vegan diet; however, there are a few differences and limitations.

Mucus, according to Dr. Sebi, is the fundamental cause of all medical conditions. He felt that problems arise when mucus builds up in the system and that they can only occur in an acid medium. Thus it's critical to consume foods that, when combined with our systems' biochemistry, provide an alkaline condition. Eating a diet from Dr. Sebi's recommended food list (see Chapter "Dr. Sebi's Approved Food List") will help the body's alkaline environment as it improves and reaches optimal health. If all of these ailments are related to mucus, inflammatory response, and acid in the system, then a slow and clogged lymphatic system is to blame.

The lymphatic system was among the most highly influential systems in the body, yet it is also one of the most overlooked. Millions of kilometers of lymphatic tubes flow interstitially across our organ systems, meaning they form in the area between and surrounding the cells. The debris of the cells is taken out by the lymph system via the channels and cleansed by the kidneys and epidermis in a fully functioning lymphatic system. Sadly, everyone seems to have a clogged lymphatic system, which prevents metabolic debris from being eliminated. Rather, when we are biologically feeble, it concentrates in our lymphatic system, producing inflammatory processes and mucous to build all over the body.

Pathogens, viral infections, and other harmful elements are carried out of the body through the lymphatic system, which promotes acidity. The cells, tissues, and glands are all deteriorating as a result of the sluggish lymphatic system. When acidic foods such as protein, dairy, and some grains (such as gluten) come into contact with our systems' biochemistry, the lymphatic system becomes blocked, acidic, and sluggish. Alkaline foods, such as strawberries, cantaloupe, and uncooked vegetables in general, are the greatest foods to consume to prevent lymphatic obstruction since they are both nourishing and astringent at the cellular level. Contaminants and blocked lymphatic fluids are drawn out from the cells, tissues, and glands with their support.

Acidity and mucus, according to Dr. Sebi, might cause a variety of disorders. For instance, pneumonia can be precipitated by the growth of mucus in the lungs. He went on to say that eating some foods and shunning others like the devil may assist the body to cleanse. It may also raise the body's alkalinity, which lowers the chance of accumulating a variety of ailments. The cells may be regenerated, and toxins can be readily eliminated by leaving the blood alkaline. Furthermore, he claims that illnesses cannot thrive in an alkaline environment. Other plant-based diets are built on his premise of making the system more alkaline. Dr. Sebi's strategy involves consuming a list of permitted foods as well as taking particular supplements. Dr. Sebi recommended that this diet be maintained continuously for the remainder of one's life in order for an individual to cure itself.

What are Herbs and Their Parts?

Herbs are generally solely the leaves, stalks, and flowers of a plant that are greenish or leafy. Medicinal plants, on the other end, such as those certified by Dr. Sebi, often employ different components of the plant, such as the root, bark, berry, fruit, and so forth. Furthermore, while many spices, such as curcumin and ginger, are often referred to as herbs, there is a distinction between the two. Numerous plants that are essentially spices, such as cinnamon, cumin, and tamarind, are commonly labeled as curative herbs, despite the fact that they are truly spices.

Healing or electric herbs are plants that aid in the healing, rebuilding, and nourishing of the human body. They are found in the environment and are alkaline. They haven't been hybridized, treated, or chemically manipulated in any way. Electrical herbs aid with enhanced brain performance by improving electrical impulses in the neurons. It improves the clarity of mind and the ability to utilize one's faculties. The human species can crawl, run, jump, and leap because of electrical impulses. There would be no mobility or existence without electricity. You should give your body electrical (alkaline) food if it is electrical in nature. Electrical herbs are not genetically hybridized, non-GMO herbs grown in the wilderness. Electric herbs are wildcrafted and cultivated without using insecticides or synthetic fertilizers.

Many plants function pharmaceutically as well as via action, giving a compelling case for their use in treatment, particularly when synthetic medications are unavailable. It's worth noting that many common synthetic medications are used to relieve symptoms and speed up the healing process. In other words, as compared to medications, natural therapies based on natural herbs will provide a comprehensive cure. Many individuals find it difficult to choose between medications and herbs since the information they need to make these decisions is usually unavailable to the public at large.

Plants are necessary for human life, irrespective of what you name them or how you define them. They not only give food, shelter, and construction materials, but they also absorb carbon dioxide and release oxygen, allowing humans to breathe. Plants also aid in the

purification of our waterways. They also nourish and heal in addition to all of this. When we think of herbs, we think of the taste they provide to our cuisine, but they also have a variety of additional functions.

1. Domestic Uses

Basil repels flies, rosemary repels mosquitos, and a blend of mashed cloves and lavender repels fish moths away from your textbooks and clothing. Raw herbs may be used to refresh your home, while dehydrated plants can be used to create a fragrance.

2. Cosmetic Uses

Herbs may help with practically any aesthetic issue, such as thinning hair, stained tooth, loose skin, and so on. They may be used to produce fragrances or infusing bath or therapeutic oils.

3. Medicinal Applications

Brew, elixir, salve, infused oil, lotion, cream, essential oil, or Bach cure are the most common herbal treatments. They are a viable option for a variety of over-the-counter medications.

4. Culinary Uses

Raw or dehydrated herbs may be added to foods or beverages, or infused oil, vinaigrette, or cream can be made.

Parts of a Plant

There are approximately 300,000 species of plants, and despite their variations in size, structure, and hue, the majority of them share certain characteristics.

1. Bark

The bark of shrubs and trees protects them from the environment. Its primary purpose is to save moisture while also protecting the plant from elevated heat, sickness, and pests. Some plants have strong enough bark to protect them from wildfires. The plant will die if the bark is severely damaged.

2. Flowers

Flowers' primary purpose is to make you want to smell and gaze at them. There would be no one to fertilize them and assure their life until they can attract pollinators, flies, or animals. Plants have vibrant colors, rich smells, and delicious nectar because of this. These factors work together to attract pollinators, who help transport pollen from one flower to another by visiting many blooms. The bloom produces seeds when fertilization has taken place.

3. Leaves

The stem's leaves are basically its organs. Respiration, or the converting of carbon dioxide, water, and Ultraviolet light into energy, is their primary activity (e.g., glucose). Those glucose molecules are converted into a variety of macromolecules that are necessary for the plant's existence. This glucose is transported to the shoots and roots via the leaflets, which helps them grow. Because sunshine and illumination are required for photosynthesis, the leaves are formed and placed in such a manner that they get the greatest amount of sun. Leaves are normally found over the soil, although certain plants, such as marine plants, have leaves that are found below or underwater.

4. Stem

stem's principal job is to transport moisture and nutrition from the bottom to the rest of the plant. Stems retain nutrients, offer support, and allow vegetative proliferation in certain plants. Certain plants, such as ginger, turmeric, and potato, have subterranean stems. Other plants produce thorny stems to defend themselves from pests. When certain plants, such as strawberries or grass, die, their subterranean stems expand and generate new plants.

5. Root

The subterranean or submerged portion of a plant is known as the root. The plant takes water and nutrients from the earth via its roots. The root also acts as a foundation, ensuring

that the plant remains stable and in one spot. There are several kinds of roots, but the taproot system is represented by primary, secondary, and tertiary roots in most plants.

Things to Remember Before Using Herbal Medicine

Herbal medications include active chemicals and are derived from plants. They may seem to be gentler than traditional drugs, but they nevertheless have an impact on your health. This implies that, although being natural, they must be consumed and prepared properly or under supervision. Before you try to treat yourself (or others) using herbal remedies, keep these eight points in mind:

- Some herbal remedies may interact with the prescription you're taking (e.g., they may reduce or enhance the effects of conventional medicine). It's advised not to use herbal remedies if you're on a prescription drug.

- If you have a significant health problem, such as liver or kidney illness, you are likely on long-term treatment and should see your physician before taking any herbal remedy. Furthermore, certain herbal remedies may interact with anesthesia and other medications. For instance, specific herbs may raise blood pressure or prevent blood coagulation, increasing the risk of blood loss during or after surgical procedures.

- You may encounter some adverse effects, such as if you have a hyper-sensitive gastrointestinal or nervous system, kidneys, skin, or other organs.

- Numerous medicinal herbs are not tightly controlled, so you use them at your own risk.

- Don't start taking medicinal plants if you are about to have a surgical procedure. Alternatively, if you are currently using an herbal medication, be sure to tell your physician.

- Pregnant or nursing ladies, as well as the aged and kids, should not use herbal remedies unless a competent healer or your physician has been contacted first.

Herbs have been used by humans for as far as they have existed. People discovered medicinal plants by accident or by a trial-and-error technique, similar to how manycreatures seek out certain plants to consume when they are ill. Sumerians recommended herbal cures for a variety of ailments as far as 5000 years ago, according to recorded archives. Herbs are beneficial because of the antioxidants and phytochemicals they carry. All plants manufacture these substances (some more than others). But, just because herbs are organic doesn't imply they're risk-free. St. John's wort and kava tinctures, for instance, are popular home treatments for emotional distress. These plants, on the other hand, may be hazardous in big doses or when combined with prescription drugs. Furthermore, several herbs, such as marijuana and coca plants, include psychotropic characteristics that have been employed for both spiritual and recreational reasons. Geological and ancient evidence show that Peruvian citizens have been using coca leaves for almost 8000 years and that marijuana was widely utilized in Asia and northern Africa as soon as the first century CE.

BOOK 2:

ALKALINE HERBES

Detoxifying Liver with Alkaline Herbs

The body contains five organs that clear toxic substances out of the blood circulation and removes them from the system in order to preserve the integrity of the physiological environment for the cells. Your liver, bowels, kidneys, skin (with its sweat and oil glands), and lungs are among these systems.

These detoxing organs, which act as exit gates for toxins in the system, are properly known as eliminatory organs. The cellular environment stays clean whenever these organs are functioning appropriately, and the generation and consumption of contaminants are not excessive. Since the excretory organs eliminate the toxic chemicals at the same pace as they develop, cells may function normally.

You may feel that your medical conditions are unavoidable and that there is little you can do regarding them, yet they are all signs of a liver that is overworked. You can repair your liver by cleaning and purifying it, removing all the impurities, lipids, and pollutants that overload it. It will help you to get clear off of all of your bothersome issues and reclaim your health and vigor. When the number of toxins is too high, however, the organs' eliminative

powers are rapidly exhausted, and the cellular environment begins to progressively amass significantly larger concentrations of toxic elements. If the excretory organs are also slow or inadequate, the pace of toxin accumulation will accelerate, resulting in disease.

In this chapter, we'll go through the importance of getting your liver detoxified with medicinal plants and herbs. Then, a subsection will highlight the consequence of having an overworked liver, i.e., all the ailments that an overburdened and slow liver creates for you. Furthermore, we'll also dive into some of the most effective medicinal herbs and herbal teas that can heal and detox your liver if consumed in appropriate amounts.

Why is Liver Detoxification Important?

In holistic medicine, cleansing of the body as a whole and of the liver especially is of paramount significance. When you understand the concept of terrain, the body's internal ecology, and naturopathic remedies, the usefulness of this therapeutic method will become clearer. For good physical health, there is a perfect terrain makeup that delivers energy and optimum endurance to the body organs. Any change in this makeup damages your wellbeing and renders you prone to sickness, which is a basic result of this desired state of things. Any alteration in the molecular terrain of the system occurs mostly as a result of chemicals that have been introduced to its optimal condition. These are compounds that are either not strange to the environment but are generally present in lesser amounts (uric acid, urea, etc.) or chemicals that do not ordinarily penetrate the terrain's makeup (preservatives, food additives, and so forth). As per natural remedies, the buildup of pollutants that overload the body's internal environment is a major cause of sickness. Overload is at the foundation of the disease, and healing necessitates the removal of these poisons.

Toxins may make us ill in a variety of ways when they build up in the system. Blood thickens, and since it is thicker and denser, it is unable to travel freely through the blood arteries. Wastes that would ordinarily be carried by the circulation to the excretory organs end up in the lymphatic system and other intracellular fluids. The longer this dirty and crowded condition persists, the more these liquids will get polluted. Toxins are detrimental because of their volume, which takes up lots of space that obstructs and blocks arteries and tissues, as well as their hostility, which irritates, inflames, and destroys cells.Certain toxins in the body are caused by tissue wear and strain. The body must constantly discard exhausted cells, red blood cell debris; utilize essential minerals, carbon dioxide, nitrogen, and other waste products. The overwhelming majority of toxins are produced through the body's utilization of dietary items. Uric acid and urea are produced by amino acids, lactic acid is produced by sugar, and a range of acids and triglycerides are produced by oils. Toxin generation is natural, and the system is capable of eliminating them. When you eat too much, the quantity of toxins in your body rises much over what is deemed acceptable. Toxic chemicals, on the other hand, should not be present in the body. Toxic chemicals are chemicals that are completely alien to normal bodily functioning and are damaging to the body. Toxic chemicals include all chemical pollutants created by contamination of the atmosphere, food, and land (lead, heavy metals, arsenic, and so on). A considerable amount of dangerous foreign compounds enter the body via typical food supplements, as well as the bulk of insecticides, pesticides, and herbicides used to protect food and livestock goods in modern farming.

Since the body is not built to accept or discharge harmful chemicals, they are hard to remove. If sickness is caused by toxins accumulating in the body, it is only natural that the best treatment would search out and remove these poisons from the body system. Emptying or purging, often known as detox, is a method of removing toxins with the aim of doing so. The liver is the organ most suited to neutralize and remove them because of its cleansing properties. The liver, like the other emunctory systems, is responsible for the elimination of a huge range of poisons. It does, however, neutralize poisons in addition to eliminating them. The other four excretory organs lack this capacity, at least not to the same degree. If they can neutralize poisons at all, it's to a very little degree. Despite the fact that the liver's job is to remove poisons and poisonous chemicals, it may get overburdened by them. As a result, the liver, more than any other excretory organ, must be in top functioning shape.

Similarly, when a patient needs to stimulate an excretory organ owing to poor physical function, the liver is usually the most suitable organ. The liver, on the other hand, takes in so much abuse when digesting poisons and poisonous chemicals that it might get overloaded. If this is the situation, and their existence in high amounts is interfering with appropriate liver enzymes, cleansing the liver becomes a primary concern in order to protect the rest of the body's health.

Ailments Caused by Liver Dysfunction

A decrease in liver function may have consequences for systems that aren't even adjacent to the liver. A quick inspection may give the idea that there is no link between the liver and the afflicted systems, but when you consider the function of the environment and chemicals in the pathogenesis of illnesses, the link becomes clear.

1. Gastrointestinal Problems

Liver dysfunction is a common explanation for constipation that is often neglected. A slow liver will not produce sufficient bile, which has the ability to promote gastrointestinal motility, the movement of food particles through the intestine. As a result, not only fiber content but also bile causes the contraction of the gut muscles. Consequently, even if there is a minor deficiency of fiber in the diet, adequate bile production allows the feces to pass through the intestines. The bowels slow down their function when there is a scarcity of bile.

The partly digested food becomes stuck and accumulates, making the gut muscles' job more difficult. Constipation will become a problem at this point. Bile also adds moisture, keeping the feces wet and smooth, making passage through the bowels easier. It prevents the feces from sticking to the mucosal surfaces of the intestinal epithelium, which are also slippery due to the presence of bile. This indicates that the stool may simply move forward. Bile deficiency, on the other end, makes feces viscous and impairs motility.

Second, the liver has a variety of functions. Bile emulsifies lipids, breaking them down into small pieces that are then targeted by the pancreatic and gut's digestive fluids. Fatty acids that have not been fully digested can induce uneasiness, bloating, and the very deep feeling that you have not digested your food if this initial step is not done properly. Furthermore, the liver aids digestion by alkalinizing the amount of food traveling through the digestive organs from the previous meal. The stomach produces very acidic digestive fluids in order to break down proteins. The pH of the food as it leaves the stomach is 2.5. The digestive and gastrointestinal fluids that are operative in the bowels, on the other hand, can only be functional in an alkaline atmosphere, i.e., when the pH is greater than 7. The liver is in charge of adjusting the pH of the meal to the level that these digestive fluids need to work efficiently. With a pH that spans from 7.6 to 8.6, the bile it produces is very alkaline. This alkalizes the food, allowing lipids to be digested completely and effectively. However, if a person has liver problems, this alkalizing action will not be enough. Fats will be poorly absorbed, resulting in a range of digestive problems.

2. Cardiovascular Diseases

Heart disease increased blood pressure, cardiac arrest, cerebrovascular disease, and other cardiovascular disorders have many different manifestations, but they all come from the same underlying cause: the buildup of fatty molecules in the circulation. The blood thickens as a result of these compounds, slowing the pace of blood flow. They produce fatty masses in the vessels when they are formed on the walls of blood vessels, diminishing their diameter and limiting blood flow. Blood coagulates when it gets too viscous and sluggish. This clot may obstruct an artery in the heart, causing a cardiac arrest, or in the brain,

causing a stroke, or anywhere else in the body, causing an embolism. However, these excess fatty compounds are chemicals that the liver might have blocked from entering the circulation if it hadn't been overburdened by a diet heavy in "poor" fats and sweets. As a result, any therapy for heart disease must include strengthening and purifying the liver.

3. Elevated Cholesterol

All of the fats we eat go straight to the liver. Only a fraction of this amount is used by the system; the rest is converted into triglycerides and cholesterol, which the liver excretes into the bile. This material next enters the bowels, where it is generally expelled with the feces if there is enough fiber (whole grain psyllium husks, natural fibers from fruit and veggies) to catch it. Fiber is necessary for the removal of cholesterol from the body. It's like a perfect trap that catches it. If there isn't enough fiber in the diet, cholesterol isn't bound and is fully absorbed by the system. Up to 90% of cholesterol may be recycled back by the gut wall and returned to the liver if you don't get enough fiber in the diet. The excess cholesterol that is reintroduced to the liver in this manner is not metabolized and removed by this organ but rather enters the overall bloodstream. It builds up in the circulation (metabolic derangement) and forms plaques on the inside of the arteries as a result of the excess amounts. The leading causes of coronary heart disease are blood viscosity and the accumulation of fatty plaques.

4. Metabolic Problems

Low blood sugar strikes certain persons on a regular basis. They experience a rapid loss of strength and vigor, as well as an overpowering sense of tiredness, which is often followed by fainting episodes and dizziness. They are frightened and nervous at times. A shortage of glucose in the bloodstream causes this lack of energy. This leads to strong and frequent cravings for sweet things like chocolate and croissants. Excessive ingestion of poor carbohydrates is the primary cause of hypoglycemia; however, the liver could also be to blame. Blood glucose is "burned" while we go about our everyday routines. Its concentration in the blood decreases, although we are usually unaware of this. The liver,

with its infinite wisdom, instantly rectifies and recovers a blood sugar rate that has gone too low. It accomplishes this by unleashing sugar into the circulation, which it has stored in the form of glycogen for this reason. When the liver is exhausted, however, the metabolism of glycogen to sugar is disrupted. As a result, the blood glucose levels drop below standard, and the liver is unable to repair it, resulting in the lack of energy that individuals experience in this condition. Cleansing the liver is, therefore, the cure. It will be able to manage blood glucose levels effectively after it has been healed and strengthened.

BOOK 3

Herbs for Liver Detox

The liver is an important organ in your body since it keeps you clear of toxic substances. It is continually processing waste that enters our system as a result of the atmosphere, nutrition, or poor lifestyle choices. Many additional health issues, including excruciating headaches, persistent exhaustion, hormone issues, nervous system abnormalities, renal problems, hepatitis, cirrhosis, and liver disease, may be caused by a liver that is no longer working effectively. Among the most efficient ways to stimulate liver function is to use herbal remedies. Hepatic plants, often known as liver drainers, are plant species used to cleanse the liver. Each one of these herbs is useful, but their actions differ widely, so it's best to switch plants throughout the duration of a lengthy therapy. This also guarantees that the system doesn't really develop a habit towards a single plant, resulting in a decreased response.

1. **Dandelion Root and Leaves**

   The vivid yellow blossoms of this well-known shrub brighten gardens and pastures. Its tall, serrated leaves give it its name. It promotes all of the liver's processes, including the creation and evacuation of bile, and is regarded as one of the finest herbs with liver-detoxing qualities by many healers. Salads made with dandelion greens are strongly advisable. For generations, the dandelion has been a well-known healing plant. It was common in ancient Egypt, Rome, and Greece, where it was widely used in traditional medicine. Dandelions were most likely brought to North America by migrants seeking therapeutic benefits. Dandelion leaves and roots may be infused for a long time, which enhances its therapeutic effects. Dandelion is a wonderful plant for liver cleaning, despite being a great coffee alternative. You may regain some vitality by detoxifying your liver. As a result, consuming it in the morning is an excellent coffee alternative that permits the whole body to remain in detox mode instead of absorbing all of the acidity that coffee use might produce. This remarkable herb has the potential to boost your immune system, eliminate free radicals, fight diabetes, alleviate nasal problems, and even fight cancer. It also boosts levels of energy, relieves stomach distress, gastrointestinal problems, gallstones, chronic stiffness, muscular pains, and dermatitis, and is used to treat viral infections. It has been used to treat viral infections and boost immunity. It helps reduce inflammation and cholesterol, lowers blood pressure, and aids in glucose homeostasis. Because of its potent antioxidant and anti-inflammatory qualities, dandelion leaf extract benefits the liver. For centuries and centuries, herbal treatments produced from dandelion root and leaves have been used to effectively treat cirrhosis and fatty liver.

2. Artichoke

The leaves of the plant, not the plant's bud, are utilized in treatment. They efficiently but gently promote bile secretion, which explains their reputation as a liver cleanser. Adults and children should consume artichoke leaves in particular. They have diuretic characteristics as well.

3. Garlic

Garlic is a great liver cleanser since it's strong in selenium and allicin. It increases the activity of liver enzymes, making it simpler for the liver to handle and eliminate pollutants. Garlic creates a number of sulfur-containing chemicals that are necessary for the body's nourishment and metabolism. Allicin and selenium, two key elements found in this plant, have been demonstrated to protect the liver from acid toxicity and help it detox.

4. Milk Thistle

The most well-known natural treatment for liver problems is milk thistle. It aids in detoxification, bile synthesis, and liver regeneration. Milk thistle is a herbaceous plant belonging to the Asteraceae family that may be found all around the Mediterranean. Milk thistle is beneficial to liver function because of its antioxidants, anti-inflammatory, cleansing, and regenerative capabilities. It regenerates liver tissues by encouraging the generation of new cells, renewing them, and preserving them from further harm. Its tonic and decongestant effects aid with tiredness, depression, and food intolerances by improving liver function. The silymarin molecule is responsible for the liver's defense. Hepatitis, cirrhosis, drinking, opioids, and environmental contaminants are all absorbed via diet, water, breath, and skin. Thus it's important to get enough of it. It also has galactogenic characteristics since it contains a lot of phytoestrogens, which increases milk production in females. Female hormone synthesis is regulated by phytoestrogens, which is important for a female's overall health.

5. Licorice

[i]Licorice has anti-hepatitis and anti-cancer properties. The licorice root is very useful for liver cleansing. Licorice is a plant that belongs to the bean family and grows as an annual herb. Since olden history, it has been appreciated for culinary and medicinal purposes throughout the Arab World, southwestern Asia, and south of Europe. Licorice's Greek name indicates "sweet root." Other licorice kinds exist, but G. glabra is the most often used in cooking. Licorice is now cultivated all over the Middle East and Central Asia, as well as in mainland Europe and the western United States. Just the roots are utilized, despite the fact that the plant produces little pods with five seeds a piece. When the plants are 3 to 4 years old, they are picked, washed, cut, and dried. Licorice sticks are made from the long segments of the roots (not to be confused with dark black licorice sticks that are actually dried concentrated licorice extract). The leftover roots are cut, diced, or crushed into a powder, and licorice extract is made from them. The powder form of licorice is light brown to grayish-green, with a brown exterior and a light tan inside. When bitten into, the roots have a scent like tobacco—licorice is often used as a flavor component in cigarettes—but produce a pleasant taste that is comparable to fennel or anise. The powder has a strong odor.

Since the Roman era, licorice root has been recommended to relieve sore throats and coughing, chewed for its sweet flavor, and made into a pleasant drink. It is essential in the candy business today, but in most places, particularly India and China, where it was well-known to herbalists hundreds of years ago, its therapeutic qualities have eclipsed its gourmet usage. Sharpened licorice root skewers are occasionally used for grilled steak in Barcelona's Basque area, incorporating it with their taste while it cooks. Alternatively, the roots may be soaked in milk or cream to form an ice cream or custard foundation. Licorice root is an anti-inflammatory that is used in Vedic medicine to treat a number of disorders ranging from digestive discomfort to liver issues, as well as to dental cleanings. Anybody with increased blood pressure, cardiovascular illness, or renal difficulties should avoid it.

6. Chicory Root

Chicory root has long been used as a traditional treatment for liver problems. It was even utilized by the ancient Egyptians to cleanse both the blood and the liver. It aids in the generation of bile, which aids in the breakdown of fat.

7. Turmeric

Curcumin, one of turmeric's most important components, increases the development of liver detoxifying enzymes.

Curcumin also kills cancerous cells in the liver and lowers lipid levels. Turmeric is a tropical root that is related to the ginger family, and the spice originates from the plant's subterranean root systems, much like ginger.

It is indigenous to India, and India is still the world's greatest grower and supplier, but it is also extensively cultivated throughout Asia, particularly in Indonesia, as well as in South America and the Caribbean. Entire clusters of turmeric plants are carefully separated from the ground, and the tiny rooted cuttings, known as fingers, are cut off from the bigger roots and cooked or steamed.

This procedure speeds up the drying process and prohibits the little clumps from growing. After that, they're dried and cleaned, with the skin removed before being powdered. Because dry roots are very rigid, professional processing is required. The most common kind of powdered turmeric is Madras turmeric, which is a brilliant yellow to orange in color. The Alleppey turmeric is believed to be of superior quality since it is deeper in hue. Both give color to whatever meal they're put to (as well as your fingers, cutting surface, and clothing).

Turmeric makes it considerably quicker for the liver to clear out contaminants when added to the diet. It also boosts bile synthesis (which helps the liver digest food), making the liver's work easier. Turmeric has been demonstrated to heal liver disease caused by alcohol intake, so have some turmeric on board for the next crazy night out. Turmeric is used in herbal remedies and is commonly used to create tea by infusing it with hot water. It's used to help with digestion and ease stomach pain. It's also thought to be a liver tonic and an anti-inflammatory substance for chronic ailments like bronchitis, and it's used as an antibacterial in topical treatments to heal wounds and burns.

8. Blue Vervain

Blue Vervain is a perennial herbaceous plant that grows to a height of 1 meter. Verbena is a European native that favors calcareous grounds. The ability to calm the nerves and muscles is among the most well-known vervain qualities. It comes in handy when you're under a lot of pressure. To get the most out of all of these qualities, brew herbal tea before going to bed. The anticonvulsant and sedative effects of blue vervain are significant. This might open up new possibilities for using this plant to treat neural conditions like seizures

in the future. Blue Vervain has a strong anti-inflammatory action, making it useful for treating terrible headaches, migraines, and sinusitis. It's also used to assist the system recover from fevers and illness by facilitating mucus clearance. It has the potential to increase the supply of breast milk in new moms. It also has cardio-protective properties, and its herbal tea, whether drank cold or as a rinse, may help to alleviate periodontal inflammation. Its essential oil possesses antiviral and antibacterial qualities that may help prevent and limit the spread of germs and bacteria, as well as certain forms of fungus.

9. Cascara Sagrada

Cascara sagrada is a tree indigenous to the Pacific coast of the United States, with populations in Chile and California, as well as Europe. Cascara sagrada is a laxative that helps you move your bowels. Based on one's tolerance and problem, it may be taken alone or in combination with other more strong substances like senna. It should only be used in rare situations of severe constipation and in circumstances when simple elimination with softer stools is required, such as hemorrhoids. The bark is very beneficial since it has a mechanical effect on the gut wall, but it should not be used for lengthy periods of time. Cascara should be used no more than twice or three times each week for a maximum of two weeks. Its impact lasts for around 8 hours, so it's best to have it before heading to bed to observe a difference in the morning.

Prolonged use of its essence is not suggested for people with digestive difficulties as well as those living with irritable bowel, liver, heart, or kidney illness since it is an herb that powerfully activates the whole digestive system. Cascara may help with digestion because of its impact on gut motility and fluids. The active compounds in its bark promote liquid and nutritional absorption, as well as liver function and bile evacuation. It's used to treat constipation, hepatitis, liver problems, and cancer, among other things. It's a colon cleanser that's said to improve the colon wall's muscle tone.

10. Yellow Dock

It's indigenous to Asia and Europe, but it's now spread all over the globe, where it's often regarded as a weed. Both the foliage and the roots have medicinal use. Cooking with leaves

is also an option. The yellow dock is used medicinally as an extract, syrup, or salve. Yellow dock root tonic is a fantastic treatment for a variety of liver issues. It promotes detoxification and increases the synthesis of bile, which benefits digestion as well as the general health of the liver. Conditions that can be resolved with yellow dock:

- Inadequate digestion
- Liver detox
- Skin disorders (like scabies)
- Inflamed nasal passages
- Rheumatism
- Scurvy
- Constipation

- Promotes bile production\s– In some African countries, warm dock leaves are used to treat inflamed nipples during breastfeeding and also pound and pulp the foliage for use as a piles treatment.

- The dehydrated root of yellow dock combined with hot water is often used as a gargle to cure laryngitis and as a mouth rinse. It is also efficacious against gum disease.

- Bowel infections (like ringworm)\s– Bacteria and fungi infections

- Jaundice

11. Moringa

Moringa has been dubbed the "wonder plant" for its many healing properties for decades. It's an all-natural immune booster with a ton of antioxidants. But, probably most importantly, moringa has been demonstrated to be helpful at liver cleansing and boosting liver function, both of which are critical for immune system function. When people's livers are inflamed, their bodies have a hard time getting rid of pollutants, reducing their immunity. Moringa, luckily, is a potent natural anti-inflammatory. Moringa has been investigated for its 40 natural antioxidants and tens of anti-inflammatory substances, which have been shown to help the liver carry out its activities without a hiccup, which is another of the significant moringa liver benefits. Enzymes must be present in full force for your liver to cleanse properly. The enzymes in diseased livers are frequently low or non-existent, preventing detoxification from taking place. Moringa, on the other hand, may stimulate the production of liver enzymes.

12. Boldo

Boldo is a shrub that grows naturally in central Chile and Peru. Boldo is well recognized in the United States as a liver stimulant and for its potential to boost bile secretion. The tea may aid in the treatment of a number of liver and gallbladder problems, including jaundice, hepatitis, and gallstones. The tea may also help with hunger stimulation, digestion, intestinal health, and bloating and constipation relief. Boldo has a distinct, somewhat bitter flavor, which, you all know, is frequently a sign of a food's healing capabilities. It may be consumed on its own or mixed with yerba mate, a famous South American beverage. Boldo's leaves carry all of the plant's therapeutic qualities. They're used to brew tea, a drug-free option that's been around since the dawn of mankind. It was originally used to treat muscular pain and achy joints. This herb is now recognized to help in the healing of liver problems, digestion, and gallbladder problems. Boldo is also found in regions that have a Mediterranean climate

Boldo tea is a diuretic that helps to reduce the development of uric acid in the blood by increasing urine frequency and amount. It also gets rid of extra salt, fluid, and bile that might otherwise build up and create problems. Peeing on a regular basis may assist in controlling blood pressure, increase hunger, promote digestion, and reduce gas production in the gastrointestinal system. Boldo tea also aids in the treatment of fatty and inflamed livers, as well as cirrhosis, hepatitis, and indigestion. Boldo tea may be used to cure a variety of conditions, including moderate dyspepsia and gastroenteritis. Boldo tea may help boost bile production from the liver during normal working circumstances. As a result, food degradation and metabolic activity in the stomach are accelerated. This guarantees that your food is processed quickly and that the amount of stagnant food in your stomach is reduced. As an outcome, you'll have fewer digestive troubles, including flatulence, cramping, and acidity. Put 1 cup of boiling hot water on 1 teaspoon of dried leaves to prepare boldo drink, steep for 10 to 15 minutes, and take three to four times per day.

Detoxifying Herbal Teas For Liver

Herbal teas have been utilized as remedies since olden history and for good motives. They're effective. They are plants having delicious and fragrant qualities that are used to enhance dishes, make teas, unwind, or treat medical conditions. Coffee, a booster of the nervous system, tannins having an astringent action, and mineral salts are all found in herbal teas. You are supposed to consume as much water as you like in addition to teas. This aids in the removal of toxic materials from the body and helps you lose weight. Liquids support liver function and, most crucially, increase urination. Try to drink as much freshwater as necessary.

1. Nettle Tea

The stinging nettle, often known as nettle, is a plant native to Northern Europe and Asia. Urtica dioica is its scientific name. The plant has lovely heart-shaped foliage and pink or yellow blooms, but the stalk is coated with small, rigid bristles that, when contacted, emit irritating compounds.

Even though the irritating characteristic of raw nettle is well-known, dehydrated nettle is among the most powerful cleansing herbs. It aids in urinary tract cleaning, and it also includes histamine, which may assist with allergy symptoms. Many plants are beneficial for

spring and summer detoxification and reducing clinical manifestations of bodily toxicity; however, nettle is an excellent option for inflammatory dermatitis and allergies, such as coughing and difficulty breathing.

2. Ginger Tea

Garlic has huge quantities of allicin and selenium, which are two distinct substances that help detoxify the liver. You may activate liver enzymes that break down and drain toxins in the body by introducing just a tiny bit of this spicy plant to your diet. Though ginger is often referred to as a root, it is really a tuber, the subterranean portion of the ginger plant's stem. Ginger is flexible in addition to having a distinct, enticing taste that is both warm and spicy. It may be prepared in a variety of ways, including fresh, dehydrated, crushed, juiced, or compressed to extract the oil. Healers have employed ginger as a natural treatment for millennia in all of these ways. Ginger is a gastrointestinal remedy that is also supposed to assist with seasickness. Ginger tea may be used to relieve a throat infection or to offer a pleasant, comforting boost, or it can be consumed before traveling.

3. Rosemary Tea

Rosemary is a Mediterranean shrub that blooms on stalks with several tiny thin leaflets that have potent choleretic (can increase bile secretion) and cholagogic characteristics. Because the effects of rosemary are so strong, therapy with this plant should be restricted to one month. Rosemary is also quite energizing and invigorating. Thus it is not suggested for those who are easily agitated. It is highly advised that you utilize it in your meals. To brew the tea, put 1 teaspoon of the leaves in each cup, steep for 15 minutes, and drink two to three cups each day.

4. Horsetail Tea

Horsetail may be found across Asia, North America, and Europe, as well as other parts of the Northern Hemisphere. Horsetail is a one-of-a-kind herb with two different stem kinds. Early in the spring season, one kind of stem emerges, resembling asparagus besides its dark hue and spore-bearing cones on top. The adult version of the plant has branching, thin, green, barren stalks and resembles a fluffy tail when it appears in the summertime. Horsetail has often been used as a diuretic for centuries (helps rid the body of excess fluid by increasing urine output). One research looked at how persons with a background of uric acid kidney disease used horsetail. Horsetail users had more diuresis than those who didn't (urine output). Horsetail contains protective qualities, according to other research, and may suppress cancer cell proliferation.

5. Birch Tea

Birch syrup is used as a traditional treatment in Nordic, Soviet, and Asian societies for strengthening immunity, combating exhaustion, curing arthritis, lowering aches and pains, and minimizing headaches. Birch tree water has also been linked to renal and hepatic cleansing. Tea prepared from the Downy birch (Betula pubescens), which grows abundantly in the Icelandic region, is very healthy and flavorful, making it ideal for everyday use. Birch tea has anti-inflammatory and diuretic properties. Birch is said to help the liver, purify the bloodstream, and treat renal disorders. It's been used to treat bladder infections. Birch is often used to treat rheumatoid arthritis of all types, as well as increasing hypertension and fluid retention development. Saponin, a harsh chemical, resin, polyphenols, tannin, and essential oils are all found in birch leaflets.

6. Bearberry Tea

Bearberry is also known as uva ursi (Arctostaphylos uva ursi). Bearberry's antimicrobial capabilities have been proven to suppress the activity of bacteria such as Escherichia coli and certain other kinds of pathogens, hence guarding against and assisting in the prevention of gastrointestinal illnesses. Because of its strong tannin concentration, it may help with diarrhea and gastroenteritis. The plant Uva Ursi was particularly popular among American Indians, and it was often utilized in ceremonies. Herbal treatment only uses the foliage, not the fruits. It was utilized by American Indians to treat bladder infections. Uva ursi was a typical therapy for bladder infections till the finding of sulfa medicines and penicillin. Soak 3 grams of crushed leaves in 5 oz. of water for Twelve hours to prepare a drink. The drink should then be strained and consumed 3 to 4 times per day.

BOOK 4:

DR. SEBI AUTO IMMUNE SOLUTiONS

Restoring Health with Medicinal Herbs

There are three illnesses we'll talk about in this chapter, i.e., pancreas, kidneys and intestinal problems. First of all, kidney stones are made up of waste products — substances that the body doesn't need. This waste is usually excreted in urine by your kidneys. If there is excess waste or there isn't sufficient water to wash it all out, it becomes a stone. These stones can be so tiny that they resemble sand or grains. The agony that these crystals cause when they are removed by the kidney may be terrible. It is frequently likened negatively to labor or anesthesia-free operation. Medical research can't explain for sure why some individuals are more susceptible to stone formation than others. However, they do run in generations, implying a hereditary susceptibility to the illness. Prolonged dehydration has also been linked to some forms of disordered eating. Kidney stones affect around one in every 15 individuals in the developed world nowadays. In certain areas, that figure is as high as one in five. Every year, upwards of a million Americans are admitted to hospitals for treatment of the disease. And what was previously primarily a male condition now impacts many females as well.

Similarly, the pancreas is another one of our very important organs, as it helps in the production of bile which helps in digesting fats and other foods. If the pancreas is not working properly due to eating a diet full of processed, acidic foods, you will start developing gastrointestinal problems like irritable bowel syndrome. Hence, the pancreas and intestines are infinitely linked with each other. So, detoxifying and healing them with natural medicinal herbs is essential for optimal health, which is what this chapter entails.

3.1 Herbs for Pancreatic Health

The pancreas is a digestive organ that generates hormones and digestive enzymes. People who have diabetes, in particular, rely on it to operate properly. Several herbs, luckily, not only preserve the pancreatic tissues against illness but also aid in its restoration if it becomes swollen, as in the instance of pancreatitis.

1. Licorice Root

The root and subterranean roots of the perennial herb called Glycyrrhiza glabra are known as licorice roots. Licorice's anti-inflammatory qualities may help alleviate the discomfort and edema associated with pancreatitis. Licorice is a good ancient treatment for decreasing inflammation of the respiratory system since it possesses antimicrobial, antibacterial, purgative, and anti-inflammatory effects. Tea, pills, and extract are all options. This plant works well in a combining solution with other plants. Licorice root has been used as a flavor enhancer, confectionery uses, and therapeutic reasons by the Greeks, Egyptians, Asians, as well as other Eastern civilizations for ages.

2. Echinacea

The numerous echinacea plants have been utilized by native groups in North America for a long period of time. The nine species of Echinacea may be utilized, but the most frequently seem to be Echinacea Angustifolia and Echinacea purpurea. Echinacea, which is strong in antioxidants, is an effective natural therapy for a variety of airway problems (e.g., bronchitis). The root extract and raw liquid of the airborne plant are by far the most

effective therapeutic forms of the herb. It's used as a complementary treatment in Germany for common cold, persistent infections of the bronchial and lower urinary system, and topically for sores that don't heal well and persistent ulcers. Its root extract is combined with other botanicals to treat influenza-like symptoms.

3. Oregano

Oregano is an effective natural therapy for high glucose levels and many other diabetes-related problems. It also offers plenty of amazing health advantages. Antioxidants including vitamins A, C, as well as vitamin K are abundant in Mediterranean oregano. Essential oregano oil is used to treat a range of diseases, and its tea may be made to relieve coughing and upset stomachs. In the Greek region, there are several distinct types, which are generally known as rigani.

4. Garlic

Garlic is beneficial to the pancreas since it lowers blood glucose levels while also stimulating insulin production in the pancreatic tissues. The kidneys are yet another vital organ for your general wellbeing. Their major job is filtering blood, which they accomplish by eliminating waste products from the system (mainly urea). They also control the amount of water and salt in the system. Progressive kidney disease, or decrease of kidney function over time, is a life-threatening disorder. Unfortunately, many individuals are completely ignorant that their kidneys are progressively deteriorating. High blood sugar and blood pressure are the primary causes of this illness.

5. Olive Leaf Extract

The pancreas will operate better if you utilize olive leaves extract (herbal extract) on a regular basis. It also relieves the discomfort and edema associated with pancreatitis and shields the pancreas from oxidative stress induced by free radicals. Your chances of pancreatic cancer will be greatly reduced if you utilize it on a regular basis.

6. Lemons

Lemons are chockfull of vitamin C and magnesium, giving a dietary boost to pancreatitis sufferers.

7. Goldenseal

Hydrastis Canadensis is the scientific name, while goldenseal has been the most popular choice. Indigenous Americans have long used it to cure skin illnesses, gastrointestinal issues, liver problems, dysentery, and eye infections. This plant is very good for diabetes patients since it aids the pancreas by reducing blood glucose levels. Its herbal medication is made from dehydrated roots. Because it is a superb organic plant that supports glowing skin, goldenseal extract is often incorporated into a variety of skin and beauty products.

Goldenseal is used to treat the flu virus and also various upper respiratory infections, congested noses, and seasonal allergies. Goldenseal is used to treat stomach discomfort and inflammation (gastritis), gastric sores, anal ulcers, colitis (intestinal inflammation), diarrhea, stomach cramps, hemorrhoids, and extreme flatulence in certain individuals. Goldenseal is available in a variety of forms, including pills, powdered, extract, and drink.

The goldenseal root, particularly when combined with Echinacea, provides several health advantages. One of the most important advantages of Echinacea and goldenseal would be that they support the immune system.

8. Gentian

Gentian root treatment helps digestion by increasing pancreatic enzyme synthesis. Hot water mixed with gentian root has also been used to relieve edema in the liver, stomach, and spleen. Gentian root is derived from plant species of the Gentiana genus, which comprises over 400 species found in the mountains of Europe, Asia, and North America. Gentian blooms appear in a range of lovely hues. However, the root is really the only part of the plant that is utilized medicinally. It's golden in color and may be processed for tablets, infusions, extracts, and tinctures. People typically combine it with water and use it externally or consume it in herbal medicine. Decrease in hunger, bloating, intestinal gas, indigestion, gastritis, acid reflux, and puking are all treated with gentian. Fever, hysteria, and excessive blood pressure are also treated with it. Gentian is used to avoid muscular cramps, cure intestinal parasites, initiate menstrual cycles, and fight pathogens, among other things.

BOOK 5:

Herbs for Kidney Health

Dr. Sebi believed in two simple but strong principles for kidney's wellbeing: drink enough water and get rid of mucus and pollutants. You must drink sufficient liquids to make up for all other deficits while still having enough to neutralize pee. In terms of toxins, changing the things that have a negative influence on your system on a daily basis will affect the makeup of your urine. A rise in what individuals ingest has been linked to kidney stones.

We must cope with more junk as our meals become more diversified. Waste passes via the kidneys and is excreted as urine. Let's look at the herbs and medicinal plants you can take for curing as well as preventing kidney disease.

1. Horsetail

It is prized for its diuretic effects, which aid in the elimination of waste from the urinary system and bladder. To manufacture medication, just the portions of the herb that are above the surface are utilized. Horsetail is used to treat "water retention" (puffiness), kidney and urethra stones, bladder infections, leakage (incapability to regulate urine), and overall kidney and bladder problems. The kidneys struggle hard to clear contaminants and control urine; horsetail may aid in this process by removing uric acid, which forms kidney stones. There is a strong link between ingesting horsetail and having reduced uric acid concentrations in the body, excess of which ultimately creates kidney stones. Baldness, hepatitis, cirrhosis, fragile nails, joint problems, arthritis, rheumatism, bone disease (reduced bone density), hypothermia, loss of weight, intense menstrual cycles, and profuse bleeding (severe bleeding) of the nasal passage, chest, or gut are also treated with it.

2. Green Tea

It is suggested to those whose kidney function is not in optimal condition because of its potent anti-inflammatory and hypotensive qualities. It also comprises antioxidants, which aim to minimize kidney stones from forming. Green tea includes catechins, which are a type of flavonoids that seem to suppress infectious diseases by attaching to the virus and thereby blocking the pathogen from reaching the host tissues. It comes in the form of tea bags or dried leaves. To make the tea, combine 20 ounces of green tea leaves with 6 ounces of water. Green tea may also be consumed as a pill or capsule three to four times each day. Consume no more than 5 cups of green tea each day.

3. Hydrangea Root

This herb is excellent for urinary and renal function. Restricts kidney stones from developing by assisting the body in using calcium so that there isn't an excess that the tissue will convert to kidney stones.

4. Couch Grass

The plant will boost your kidney output (peeing), which can help you cure any of the urinary tract infections simply since the more and more you pee, the more microbes you will clear out. Couch grass may also aid in the removal of kidney stones.

5. Goldenrod

Goldenrod, which is also known as Solidago canadensis, has traditionally been used to treat sores on the body. It's also been used as a purgative, which means it aids in the removal of surplus water from the system. In Europe, it's used to cure urinary tract infections and kidney problems, as well as to minimize or cure them. Goldenrod is often used in infusions to assist in washing away kidney stones and prevent urinary tract illnesses. "To make complete" is the meaning of the term solidago. It's a long-used treatment for bladder and kidneys and renal ailments in general. Goldenrod is sometimes used as "irrigation treatment." This is a treatment that entails consuming goldenrod with plenty of water to enhance the flow of urine in order to cure chronic conditions of the lower urinary tract and also kidney and urinary tract stones. Its usage as a bladder and kidneys health defender is also supported by new research.

6. Chanca Piedra

Chanca piedra often referred to as "stone buster," is a medicinal herb that is supposed to be a miracle cure for kidney diseas Chanca piedra is a Phyllanthaceae family annual herb. The plant may be found in the Amazon jungle as well as in other tropical climates across the globe. An herbal remedy made from the whole plant is utilized as infusions, pills, liquid solutions, and capsules. Gout recurrences are caused by the growth of uric acid in the vascular system, which also causes kidney stones. Chanca piedra has been proven to help regulate this excessive production of uric acid and avoid painful gout episodes. The plant is said to help with ulceration, kidney and bladder stones, and a variety of disorders involving the kidneys, liver, and gastrointestinal tract. When it relates to effectively removing kidney stones, it's the most popular plant in South America. Chanca piedra got its name from its usefulness as a renal stone remedy. The herb's alkaline qualities may aid in the prevention of gallbladder and toxic kidney stones.

7. Java Tea

Drinking Java tea would not only enable you to keep your kidneys functional, but it will also certainly assist you in disintegrating kidney stones and healing renal infections.

8. Dandelio

Dandelion root is a powerful cleanser and an excellent herbal renal detoxifier. Dandelion is a popular blooming plant that grows all across the globe and is prized for both its roots and blooms. As a diuretic and purgative, dandelion is commonly used with the burdock plant to treat gastrointestinal diseases. It relieves upset stomach and gas while also improving the efficiency of the liver and gallbladder as well as intestinal health. Its diuretic effect is mild on the body due to its mineral content, which partly refills the amount lost via peeing, allowing the person to maintain a healthy alkaline equilibrium. It may help ladies with fluid retention. Dandelion is also great for the cure of urinary tract infections and kidney problems. Its anti-inflammatory properties aid healing while also safeguarding renal function. It may be used on the skin to treat dermatitis, wounds, and scars, as well as to enjoy its anti-aging properties. It helps with skin pigmentation problems. Finally, it aids in blood sugar management, making it a viable alternative for diabetics.

9. Celery Root

Both the root and the seeds are diuretic and should be used by anybody who has urinary tract issues. Dr. Sebi and Kidney Disease

By eliminating extra compounds that may make your blood more acidic or alkaline, your kidneys assist in controlling the pH level (acid concentration) in your blood. Low pH blood is considered acidic and may result in potentially fatal medical conditions. With renal disease, your kidneys have a harder time removing acid from your blood. Because of this, persons with kidney illness may benefit from eating an alkaline-rich diet low in acidic foods. Your doctor could sometimes prescribe drugs to aid with this balance.

5.1 Acidic vs. Alkaline

Your diet may impact how much acid is in your blood. Foods that contribute to acidity range in pH from 0 to 7, whereas alkaline foods range from 7 to 14. Eat exactly the portions of these acidic items that your nutritionist or physician advises you to boost your diet's alkaline content:

Acidic Foods

•   Grains and grain products; Meat; Poultry; Fish; Cheese; Egg Yolk; Peanuts; Carbonated beverages, particularly cola.

•   Additionally, consume these alkaline foods in the quantities your dietician or physician advised.

Alkaline Meals

•   Legumes, egg whites, textured soy protein, fruits (lower potassium options if you're on a low-potassium diet), and vegetables (lower-potassium choices if you are on a low-potassium diet)

5.2 Eat Your Fruits and Veggies

Your pH levels may be better balanced by eating more fruits and vegetables and other high-alkaline foods. More fruits and vegetables in the diet are generally not a problem for patients with the early-stage renal disease since they typically do not need to restrict their potassium intake. But those with advanced renal disease often need to restrict their potassium consumption. To maintain low potassium levels and maintain pH balance, it is important to consume low-potassium fruits and vegetables.

5.3 Talk to a Dietitian

Each body is unique. To ensure you're receiving the necessary nutrients for your body, speak with your nutritionist and the renal care team before making any dietary adjustments.

BOOK 6:

dr sebi approved Herbes

Herbs for Intestinal Detox (Colon Cleanse)

Colon cleansing is a term used to describe the process of removing waste from the intestines. For hundreds of years, it has been a common practice. But, while an intestinal detox has numerous advantages, it also has some drawbacks. Herbs in the shape of brews, pills, or powders are a substitute for colon cleansing in a facility. Many plants are anti-inflammatory and function as herbal laxatives.

1. Cascara Sagrada

Cascara sagrada is a plant indigenous to the Pacific coast of the United States, with populations in Chile and California, as well as Europe. Its skin is the most helpful component, and it is so potent that it requires a year after collecting to nearly fully eliminate the side effects of its usage. After that year, it may be used for a variety of ailments without causing stomach discomfort, vomiting, or diarrhea. It's a mild laxative that helps you move your bowels. Based on one's tolerance and problem, it may be taken alone or in combination with other more strong substances like senna. It should only be used in rare situations of severe constipation and in circumstances when simple elimination with soft stools is required, like hemorrhoid

The bark is very beneficial since it has a mechanical effect on the gut wall, but it should not be used for lengthy periods of time. Cascara should be used not any more than twice or three times each week for a maximum of 15 days. Its impact lasts for around eight hours, so it's best to apply it before getting in bed to observe a difference in the morning. Excessive use of its extract is not suggested for anyone with digestive difficulties or even those living with irritable bowel, liver, cardiovascular, or renal problems since it is an herb that powerfully activates the whole digestion process. Cascara may help with digestion because of its impact on gut motility and hydration. The active compounds in its bark promote liquid and nutritional uptake, as well as liver function and bile output. It usually causes a bowel movement within ten to 12 hours. Therefore it's wise to take it at nighttime so you can use the toilet more easily in the morning.

2. Senna

Senna tea or pills are a strong laxative that shouldn't be taken for any more than a couple of days at a time.

3. Rhubarb Root

The word "rhubarb" originated from the Latin word "rhabarbarum." The roots of Rhabarbarum were employed as a cleanser by the Chinese as way back as five thousand years ago. Rhubarb is an herb that is indigenous to Asia and Europe which is now grown all over the globe. For generations, its root has also been used to treat many ailments. It's harvested when the plant is about a year old, dried, and used in tiny pieces or powdered, mostly in teas. Rhubarb root is taken as a laxative, as well as to enhance liver function and digestion. Since it has a strong impact on your bowels, it is important to keep its usage to a minimum in terms of amount and regularity. Rhubarb root includes numerous chemicals

that assist digestion by activating the gall bladder and cleansing the blood by removing heavy metals. It also helps in the detoxification of toxic chemicals and dangerous microorganisms from the intestine. Constipation, gas, and cramping may all be relieved with this supplement.

4. Psyllium Husk

Psyllium seeds and husk are a very well-recognized colon cleaning folk medicine. The presence of mucilage, a form of fiber that absorbs moisture in the gastrointestinal tract, is what gives it such an effective laxative effect.

5. Fennel.

Fennel is a fragrant plant indigenous to the Mediterranean region that comes from the Umbelliferae family and has the scientific name Foeniculum Vulgare Miller. Fennel is primarily used as a fragrant plant, but it also offers a wide range of health advantages. Purifying and gastrointestinal herbal teas may be made using leaves and seeds. The seeds, in particular, are high in active substances, which are beneficial to the biological mechanisms of the gastrointestinal tract. Its crude extract is likewise high in estrogen-like chemicals. It is often used in conjunction with laxatives, such as rhubarb or senna. It's gentle to administer to kids on its own. It also has an antispasmodic action, which aids in the elimination of unpleasant digestive colic in infants, and is ideal for individuals experiencing abdominal discomfort as a result of digestive problems.

Fennel is a diuretic that aids in the removal of excess bodily fluids. Its cleansing characteristics make it even better when combined with other alkaline plants, including dandelion root and milk thistle. Fennel tea has several health advantages, particularly for individuals who suffer from digestion problems such as stomach ache, abdominal discomfort, stomach pain with contractions, and gastritis with reflux may all profit greatly from a decent cup of fennel tea, which can be consumed following dinners or throughout the day to cleanse the stomach. Fennel improves stool motion, removes excess gas, sanitizes the colon, and relieves cramping and aches in cases of gastrointestinal abnormalities, inflammatory bowel disease, constipation, diarrhea, spasms.

Fennel has a purgative effect, which helps to clear and remove mucus. In the night, a warm infusion promotes respiration and helps you get a good night's sleep.

6. Barberry Bark

This plant promotes bile production and works as a natural laxative, which benefits intestinal function.

7. Black Walnut

Juglans nigra is the official name for the tree, which is predominantly found in the United States of America. The seed is the only part of the plant that may be eaten. They're a potent

natural vermifuge and are used to fight intestinal worms that may harm people. Candida Albicans is a fungal pathogen in our intestines. Consuming black walnuts will improve our intestinal health and help Candida Albicans' life as difficult as possible.

BOOK 7:

Boosting Immune System with Alkaline Plants

Regardless of the severity of an illness, even deadly viruses like Ebola, some individuals stay healthy while being infected. In reality, clinical investigations have repeatedly demonstrated that most people's bodies contain pathogenic bacteria, even if they never get sick. Numerous studies have indicated that the stronger your immune response is, the less probable you are to contract an illness and, when you do, the milder your illness will be. This is especially correct when it comes to infections like Lyme. Researchers have long known that the greater particular immune indicators are, the less probable disease is to develop, and if it does, the sickness will be milder than when the immunological indicators are weak. In reality, our immune response is our first line of protection. Its mission is to keep us healthy and, if sickness does strike, to correct it. As a result, the first and most crucial aspect of health and strength is a strong immune system.

In this chapter, we'll outline a number of medicinal herbs and plants that you can use to boost your immune response.

4.1 Immunity Boosting Herbs

In reality, our immune response is the primary line of security. Its mission is to keep us healthy and, if sickness does strike, to remove it. As a result, the first and most crucial aspect of health and strength is a strong immune system. When it pertains to improving, healing, or optimizing the immune system, a few herbs are noteworthy. They may all be taken for a long time and have few adverse effects. While some of these plants are effective against specific illness microorganisms, their real power comes from their ability to boost different parts of the immune response, providing protection against poisons and illness for certain organs and tissues. They protect the body against the impact of stress and boost the body, particularly the immune response, to better cope with negative situations, whether internally and externally present.

1. **Elderberry**

   have been utilized for a variety of diseases since the late 1700s. Northern Africans and medieval Asians utilized it extensively to treat a variety of ailments. Healers use it medicinally to enhance the immune response throughout the winter and flu seasons. Almost every component of the elderberry plant may be used medicinally or in cooking. Dr. Sebi emphasized berries since research has shown that they contain antioxidants and have anti-diabetic, anti-inflammatory, immune-modulating, and antidepressant effects. It is also reported to have anti-cancer effects. They assist in detoxing the body, enhance eyesight, accelerate the body's metabolism, enhance lung health, lessen inflammatory processes, and fight against chronic illness since they are high in antioxidants. Elderberry loosens phlegm in the respiratory system and airways, making it much easier to cough up phlegm and preventing pneumonia or bronchitis.

It may be cooked or may be used to produce juice, jellies, flavorings, wine, cocktails, and appetizers. The most common method is to create a syrup out of it or to use it as an infusion or drink. If you are unable to consume the plant, it may be taken in tablets or capsules, generally three pills each day. Two to four times a day, consume one or two teaspoons of concentrated liquid extract.

2. Ashwagandha

Ashwagandha is a species indigenous to India's dry areas that have spread to northern Africa and the Mediterranean, mainly the mild, semi-arid settings with enough rainfall in the monsoon season. Although the plant is not widely cultivated (or recognized) in the United States, it is a widespread agricultural species in its native area. Tuberculosis, malnutrition in kids, gout, general loss of function, nervous stress, mental confusion, memory problems, lack of muscular activity, and spermatorrhea have all been treated with it. Its main purpose is to re-energize a body that has been worn down by long-term systemic sickness or advanced age.

3. Licorice

Licorice is a good folk treatment for decreasing inflammation of the lung tissue since it possesses antimicrobial, antiviral, purgative, and anti-inflammatory effects.

4. Nopal

The nopal cactus is native to the American Southwest and Mexico's deserts. It really is a ubiquitous component in Mexican cooking, but it's meant to be eaten raw while the fruit is still luscious and soft. Jam, stews, soups, and appetizers are all made using nopal fruit. Antiviral and antioxidant activities are at the heart of the nopal's curative benefits. In

Mexico, there are approximately 100 species of nopal, and it's been used in indigenous medicine for centuries. It protects against viral diseases. Antiviral qualities have been discovered in nopal cactus, and preliminary research suggests that it may be used to treat herpes simplex, respiratory infections, and HIV/AIDS. It also helps to keep nerve fibers safe. You may experience sensory impairment or discomfort if your nervous system cells are destroyed. The nopal cactus may help to prevent this. It also guards tissues and organs against free radicals. Because nopal is abundant in antioxidants, it defends your cells from free radical damage.

5. Guaco

Guaco often spelled huaco, is the popular name for a group of plants classified as Mikania guaco that may be located in South America's rainforests. Guaco was used by the rainforest tribes for millennia to treat cobra and bug bites. The leaves are cooked into a brew that may be consumed or powdered into a mixture that can be used to treat an exterior wound. It may also be used to cure itchiness on any other inflamed skin or rashes as tea. Bronchodilators are substances that widen the breathing passages in the chest that are used to treat viral infections of the chest, pneumonia, and other respiratory ailments. It's also an expectorant (tends to help in clearing mucus) and a cough reliever, which is the reason it's used to treat a variety of upper respiratory illnesses like colds, influenza, and pneumonia.

6. Astragalus

It's also referred to as milk vetch or huang qi. It's derived from a legume or bean. Even though there are other species of this plant, astragalus membranaceus is included in the majority of astragalus pills. The plant is reported to provide a variety of health advantages, particularly those for the cardiovascular system. The immune system seems to be stimulated by astragalus. It possesses antioxidant properties that prevent the generation of free radicals. Oxidative stress destroys tissues and organs and is connected to a variety of aging-related health issues. It is beneficial to the body in combating physiological,

psychological, and emotional turmoil. It is mostly used to treat the wart-causing Human papillomavirus (HPV). Quinovic Acid Glycosides are found in it, and they help to defend the body's immunological system. The herpes virus is treated using this herb.

7. Chaparral

Chaparral, also known as Larrea, is a plant that grows mostly in Mexico and the United States of America and is well-known for its fragrant blooms. Chaparral may help to clear mucus from the airways, which can help with pneumonia and bronchitis. The lymphatic system and blood are cleansed off of toxic substances as a result of its cleansing function. Chaparral has also been used to combat sexual problems for years. Currently, it's most recognized for its capacity to keep the body alive while it's sick from malignancies, particularly those of the skin, stomach, and liver.

8. Bladderwrack

Bladderwrack may be found along the western Baltic Sea, North Sea, Pacific, and Atlantic Ocean shores. It's rich in iodine, which is essential for thyroid function. It may be used to enhance immune function and increase energy. Bladderwrack may be eaten whole, made into tea, or combined with marine turtles in drinks and shakes. To brew tea, mix 1 teaspoon each mug of hot spring water, then set aside for fifteen minutes before sipping. This might be used once or twice a day.

9. Chamomile

The herb is native to Europe, and it has been used for medical reasons for ages. It was adored by the ancient Egyptians because of its remarkable healing properties. It has a relaxing impact on the skin and a relaxing impact on the mind. This is why it is used to treat skin ailments or as a tea to aid sleep. Chamomile enhances your immune response by assisting you in getting a good night's sleep since your immune system operates best when you've rested enough. It has a powerful soothing effect, so prepare a powerful brew prior to going to bed if you're having difficulties sleeping. To treat sunburn, cleanse your face with chamomile tea or soak in a bathtub with strong chamomile tea. Never ever use teabags; always use loose chamomile.

10. Irish Sea Moss

It's a kind of seaweed that grows along the coasts of Europe and America. It dwells in the deep end, where daylight is scarce, and rose to fame in the mid-1800s when it helped feed Irish people during a terrible starvation phase. Irish Sea Moss contains a gel that has antioxidant and anti-inflammatory properties and may be used for a variety of ailments, including herpes. Herpes is a disease that goes unnoticed in the body until it manifests itself in the form of painful sores. Sea moss gel may help to heal wounds and maintain healthy skin. Sea moss fibers help to improve intestinal health, which leads to a stronger immune system. It also lowers cell damage, which helps prevent mental impairment and diseases such as Parkinson's and Alzheimer's.

11. Reishi

The Asian word for the herb, reishi, is now the most popular term for the plant in the Western world. The active elements in the red reishi fungus, which is the best version available, include water-soluble polysaccharides, beta-glucans, and hetero-beta-glucans. These polysaccharides help to strengthen the immune function, combat cancer, and reduce high blood pressure. A specific a protein found in reishi also helps to enhance immune function. Reishi supplementation is generally believed to be harmless, although individuals

receiving organ donations or other immunosuppressive treatments ought to be cautious since any immune-modulating agent might interfere negatively with other medications

12. Rhodiola

Rhodiola rosea is a unique herb with a long and diverse background of use. It is considered to boost the neurological system, combat depression, boost immunity, raise exercise performance, improve cognitive function, promote weight loss, promote sexual performance, and boost energy levels. It's been recognized for a long time as a powerful adaptogen. Adaptogens are chemicals that assist in regulating biological functioning by increasing the body's general resilience.

Its brew has long been used in Central Asia as the most efficient local therapy for respiratory infections. Tibetan healers use it to treat tuberculosis and tumors. Traditional Tibetan medicine uses the herb to promote blood flow and relieve congestion. Although there are signs of its usage as far back as the late 1700s in Nordic nations, the herb was never a big therapeutic herb. Antifungal and antibacterial properties have been discovered in a variety of Rhodiola. Rhodiola kirilowii, for example, is effective for the hepatitis C virus. It defends cells against tert-butyl hydroperoxide damage and boosts the immune system's response. Furthermore, it activates the natural immune system and has powerful immunogenic effects. Central Asians believed that a tea made from Rhodiola rosea was the most efficient remedy for colds and influenza. It was administered by Mongol experts for TB and carcinoma.

13. Prodigiosa

Prodigiosa is a Californian shrub. It is typically used to cure many ailments. Prodigiosa is one of the most often utilized herbs to treat diabetes. Its hypoglycemic impact lowers blood glucose levels while also stimulating stomach juices, bile production, and gallbladder cleansing. It's a good plant for females because of its modest anti-inflammatory impact on the urinary tract and mild menstrual stimulating properties.

14. Thyme

Thyme contains antibacterial, antiviral, and antimicrobial activities. Thus it may assist with practically any breathing problem. It may be consumed as a drink or a potion, but it's most effective when taken as a crude extract.

15. Kalawalla

They originate in the Honduran rainforests and bloom solely on palm trees in a synergistic bond. It contains antioxidants, which aid in the immune system's strengthening. It is used as a blood cleanser by the native population. It includes three different kinds of amino acids, all of which are potent antioxidants that shield your DNA from damage caused by free radicals. Kalawalla is very beneficial for persons with skin diseases, and it's also been used to treat brain illnesses such as Parkinson's.

16. Echinacea

Echinacea, which is strong in antioxidants, is an effective natural therapy for a variety of breathing difficulties (e.g., bronchitis).

17. Boneset

Eupatorium perfoliatum is a plant that has a rich tradition of being used to treat viruses and flu. Boneset was also employed by American Indians for the cure of musculoskeletal aches, as well as the repair of fractured bones. Some of the first applications of boneset were as potions or skin band-aids. Using the plant as a brew or drink did not become popular until the mid-nineteenth century. The herb's popular name, boneset, comes from its power to alleviate the dreadful fevers that come with flu.

BOOK 8:

Dr. SEBI TREATMENTS

Heal Infections and Viruses with Alkaline Herb

Perhaps no technical breakthrough has been more extensively publicized and exploited than the discovery of antibiotics. The effectiveness of the scientific approach over untrained treatment in history is often recognized as one of the key successes of the power of scientific and contemporary healthcare in Western society. There are several reasons why individuals nowadays switch to herbal medications, particularly antivirals, but you must ensure that the decision is good for you. According to research, over one-third of Americans take herbal treatments and want to keep doing so, but everyone should be aware of these risks. First, other drugs you're taking could be affected, so talk to a doctor to be sure there won't be any unwanted side effects. Second, while herbal treatments have fewer potential adverse effects than traditional antibiotics, you should still be informed of what can happen. The third point to consider is that herbal remedies are not supervised in the same way that modern medicines are. There are many tools and data given to help you make your own judgments. However, certain populations haven't been well examined, such as pregnant or nursing ladies, toddlers, or old people. It's right to always consult your physician beforehand. On the brighter side, herbal antivirals are widely available. They do not even have to be in capsule form to be effective. In fact, incorporating antiviral foods into your daily regimen is an excellent approach to help protect yourself against infections. In this chapter, we'll take a look at various herbs that have antiviral, antifungal and antibacterial properties.

5.1 How Do Herbal Antivirals Work?

It's challenging to make an effective and safe medication antiviral medicine that doesn't harm the tissue that the virus is using to proliferate. In the 1960s, trial-and-error research techniques were used to generate the very first prototype antiviral medications, which first targeted the herpes virus. Researchers couldn't figure out the correct compounds to stop viruses from reproducing till the 1980s when the whole genomic sequences of viruses became known. Antiviral medications act by preventing the virus from replicating biochemically.

Pros of Herbal Antivirals

Herbal antivirals have fewer adverse effects, are much less expensive, and are more readily accessible.

Cons of Herbal Antivirals

Because herbal antivirals are not regulated, it might be hard to get all of the facts you want. Additionally, they have the potential to interfere with other medications you're using.

5.2 Plants with Antibiotic and Antiviral Properties

Here is a list of plants that have been proven to heal viral infections and boost immune response.

1. Cloves

Cloves are a hugely appreciated spice that is well-known for their culinary and medicinal properties all across the globe. They're the "flower buds" of an Indonesian evergreen rainforest tree. Sygizium aromaticum is the official name for the spice that comes from the Myrtaceae family and the genus Sygyzium. The flower buds start off pale, then become green before maturing into vibrant clove blooms by the moment they're ready to be harvested. Buds are usually pulled up when they achieve a height of 1.5-2 cm.

2. Lemon balm

Lemon balm is a relaxing plant that is a part of the mint family. Melissa officinalis is the scientific name for this plant, which has been used for generations to relieve anxiety, improve sleep, and alleviate gastrointestinal problems. Experts have studied lemon balm and discovered that it has several health advantages. Lemon balm is a plant that originated in Europe but is now spread all over the globe. It's often used to attract pollinators, which assist in fertilizing the remainder of the crop. The plant may grow to have a height of two feet and produces bright yellow blooms where the leaflets join the stem. The leaves resemble fresh basil leaves in structure and have a lemon-like acidic and sweet aroma. The Romans and Greeks employed this plant to heal bug bites and stings. Insects dislike the sharp sour scent that the leaves emit. It has essential oils that deter insects. The essential oils generated by the leaves are often used to alleviate sleeplessness, anxiety, and uneasiness. Terpenes, tannins, and eugenol are all found in it, and they have a powerful relaxing and antiviral impact. Lemon balm is most often used to treat herpes. You should not take more than 80mg each day for more than 4 months.

3. Cat's Claw

Uncaria Tomentosa, a novel botanical nutrient, has been dubbed the Wonder Plant from Peru's Tropical Rainforest by many. It has sparked the curiosity of advocates of alternative medical treatment. The medicinal properties of this Peruvian plant have been examined at research organizations in Peru, Austria, Germany, England, Hungary, and Italy ever since the 1970s, despite being relatively unknown in the United States till lately. According to these investigations, the plant may help with osteoarthritis, tendonitis, infections, diabetes, immune disorders, chronic fatigue, cancer, herpes, major depression, irregular menstrual cycles, and stomach and intestinal issues. It has Quinovic Acid Glycosides, which support the immunological system of the body. The herpes virus is treated using Cat's Claw. Taking 60–100mg per day is safe to use.

4. Juniper

Juniper (Juniperus communis) has antimicrobial, antiviral, diuretic, and antibacterial characteristics that make it useful for treating a number of internal and exterior ailments. It was used as a therapy for viral disorders and also for childbirth in the past. Juniper is a kind of evergreen tree that may be found growing wild in Europe, Asia, and America. Though there are several types of juniper, Juniperus communis is the most prevalent in the United States. This tree may reach a height of 10 feet and has thread leaflets and seed cones. The dark scales that emerge from the cones of the juniper plant are described as berries, although they are really the therapeutic portions of the species. The male juniper's scales mature in 1.5 years, whereas the female juniper's scales mature in two to three years. It includes a compound called amentoflavone, which stops viral infections from replicating. Juniper is used to treat viral gastritis. You may consume 20–100mg of the essential oil or 2–10g of the berries.

5. Ginseng

There are **3** distinct herbs usually referred to as 'ginseng'; Korean or Asian ginseng (Panax ginseng), Siberian ginseng (Panax quinquefolius) and American ginseng (Panax quinquefolius). While it has several of the same qualities as the previous two herbs, it is no real ginseng. Panax ginseng was traditionally used to improve the gut and airways, soothe the mind, and boost general vigor in Chinese Herbal treatments. It is classified as an adaptogen, meaning that it helps to regulate and reinforce the body under stressful conditions. It's included in a lot of energy beverages and vitamins that help with energy, mental sharpness, and overall fitness. Ginseng is said to have antitumor and anti-inflammatory properties. However, there is proof that Panax can aid immunity, particularly in the case of respiratory infections. It includes ginsenosides, which have a variety of effects on the body, including improving stress tolerance and increasing vitality. Ginseng is most often used to treat flu. You should only take 2g per day and not for more than 3 months at a time.

6. Sage

Sage, like oregano, lavender, rosemary, thyme, and basil, is a Mediterranean herb that belongs to the Lamiaceae (mint) genus, which also includes thyme, lavender, rosemary, oregano, and basil. The plant has grey foliage up to 2.5 inches long (6.4 cm) and blue, violet, pink, or white blooms.

Sage is frequently used as a perfume in detergents and creams due to its distinct pleasant perfume. Sage is often used in healthcare to treat digestive issues as well as cognitive diseases, including Parkinson's and depression. Tannins and flavonoids are antiviral compounds. Sage is typically used to treat flu, but it is also effective against the herpes virus. It is made in the form of a pill, an ointment, or a culinary herb. A spoonful of crushed or raw sage in boiling hot water may be used to make a tea. Pour a quart of boiling hot water over a bunch of leaves and let it simmer overnight to make a tonic. Consume 1–2.5 g 3 times per day.

7. Garlic

Garlic has been farmed for over 5000 years, and its therapeutic benefits have been appreciated since the time of the ancient Egyptians. In very many civilizations, it is utilized as a traditional cure to prevent the common cold and flu. Garlic has been discovered to have antiviral, antibacterial, and antifungal effects in clinical examinations. Garlic's antiviral and anti-inflammatory benefits are due to its dozens of helpful components that act together. Allicin, which is responsible for garlic's strong odor, is by far the most important of them. When raw garlic is sliced or eaten, another component called allicin is created, and it may also be gotten through powdered garlic pills containing allicin capabilities. Other sulfur compounds produced by allicin include ajoene, allyl sulfides, and vinyldithiins. Due to the existence of Sallylcysteine, old garlic preparations may have some antimicrobial action. Raw garlic, allicin, and several other sulfur elements in garlic eradicate the common cold virus, numerous seasonal influenza strains, and herpes virus subtypes 1 and 2 in lab experiments. This sulfur component is most often used to combat the common cold virus.

8. Acacia

Acacia trees have mostly been prized for their extraordinary hardwood, therapeutic benefits and ornamental purposes for countless generations. Acacia was regarded as a holy wood by the Jews, and there's also a tale that Christ's crown of spikes was crafted with acacia. Acacia has grown more famous for its medicinal benefits in recent years, with many healers recommending it as an herbal cure for a number of ailments.

9. Burdock Root

Ancient healers in China, India, and Europe utilized them to ease pain and cleanse the bloodstream. Burdock is now fairly prevalent in North America and Australia, and the roots and leaves are utilized for their medicinal properties. Dr. Sebi focused his efforts mostly on roots, which are far more potent. They are harvested before blossoming and dried before being used. Burdock root may be utilized in a variety of internal and exterior treatments. Because of its high sulfur content, external usage helps combat bacterial infections, alleviate arthritis, and strengthen and cleanse hair. Burdock Root extract helps with menopausal symptoms, including hot flashes, night time sweats, irregular heartbeat, and promotes vaginal lubrication, among other things. It also aids with detoxification, blood sugar regulation, and digestion. A Burdock drink may aid weight loss by increasing

metabolic activity, decreasing hunger, and boosting a slow thyroid. Burdock root contains trace amounts of all the minerals found in the human body. It assists with dyspepsia, joint discomfort, liver detoxification, and hormone balance. Aids in the improvement of skin texture, the reduction of inflammation, and the reduction of blood sugar levels.

10. Sanguinaria (Bloodroot)

Sanguinarine is a plant alkaloid found in Sanguinaria canadensis and Poppy fumaria species' roots. It's a cationic compound that changes from an iminium ion to an alkanolamine at a pH higher than seven. The active components in most sanguinaria preparations include sanguinarine and a couple of additional alkaloids. Antibacterial, anti-inflammatory, and antioxidant activities have been discovered in this plant. It's been used to minimize plaque and tartar, and gum irritation as an antibacterial mouthwash and a toothpaste addition. It contains the alkaloids sanguinarine and berberine, which are antiviral. Sanguinarine is mainly used in the treatment of HIV infection. You may take 10-30 drops of it as a tincture once or twice a day.

11. Jacaranda

The jacaranda grows in April in Mexico, signifying the beginning of springtime. The jacaranda is a plant that originated in Bolivia and Argentina and is now grown as a

decorative plant all over the globe. Because of its stunning and long-lasting blue petals, Jacaranda mimosifolia is a subtropical plant indigenous to South and Central America that has been extensively planted abroad. The tree has been used to cure hepatitis, and the tree's petals, leaves, and trunk have been used to cure neuropathy and varicose veins in fables. Jacaranda has been clinically demonstrated to have anti-leukemia properties. Jacaranda leaf washes are used to cure injuries and skin problems, and the tree is also used to cure acne. It is effective in the treatment of infectious diseases, gonorrhea, and syphilis. Because nearly a third of the planet's population is intolerant to penicillin, the principal antibiotic used to treat this and other illnesses, having the choice provided by the jacaranda Mimosifolia is advantageous.

Glutamic acid and antibacterial oils may be found in its fruits. The utilization of jacaranda to preserve food in lieu of other preservatives has also been investigated. Nerve impingement, varicose veins, pimples, sores, leukemia, and dermatitis are all treated with it. As a result, its extract of leaves may be used topically to treat wounds or blisters caused by sexual infections. The antimicrobial activity of Jacaranda mimosifolia leaf extracts towards Bacillus cereus, and E. coli is greater than that of regular antibiotics. Staphylococcus aureus is also affected by the extract.

12. Eucalyptus

Eucalyptus is an old tree species that has been prized for its medicinal benefits for generations. Its name comes from the Greek language. It possesses expectorant and anti-inflammatory qualities, allowing mucus to be removed from the body, particularly via the respiratory system. As a result, it is used for colds, coughing, rhinitis, and pneumonia. Its essential oil contains antibacterial properties, making it beneficial in cases of candida, herpes, and cystitis. Eucalyptus may be used to treat breakouts, acne, and burns on the skin, as well as hair. It may also help with gastrointestinal problems such as ulcers, colitis, and cramping. Eucalyptus essential oil contains antibacterial and antimicrobial characteristics that may help with urinary tract disorders, including cystitis, leucorrhoea, and yeast. Eucalyptus products have a powerful antibacterial effect that helps to heal skin

conditions and soothe burns. It's great for cleaning oily scalps and hair while also restoring luster.

13. Cumin

Cumin, like parsley, is a yearly plant native to the Arabian Peninsula, while other accounts claim it started in the Nile River valley. Cumin has a long tradition of being used in cooking, dating back to 5000 BC. It was employed in fossilization by the ancient Egyptians, and it is recorded both in Old and New Testaments. It was also supposed to promote love and faithfulness. It is now grown across the Middle East and North Africa, with Iran, India, Turkey, and Morocco being leading suppliers. Cumin is picked after the seeds have matured and the stems have shriveled completely. Its essential oil has antifungal effects, according to modern medicine.

14. Black Seed

For generations, the seeds of this annual blooming plant known as Nigella Sativa have been treasured for their medicinal powers. While it was formerly known as Roman coriander, black sesame, black cumin, black caraway, and onion seed in many countries, it is now largely recognized as black seed, and it is at the very minimum an appropriate descriptor of its physical attributes. It was first cultivated and used in Egyptian civilization, according to records. In reality, black seed oil was discovered in an ancient pharaoh's crypt many decades ago. Black cumin is regarded as a healing plant in Arab traditions, which means "blessed seed." It is also claimed that the Muslim prophet Muhammad (PBUH) stated that it is "a cure for all illnesses other than death."

15. Ginkgo Biloba

Ginkgo biloba, often referred to as Maidenhair, is the world's longest-living plant species, dating back approximately 300 million years. The Asians have utilized the herb in folk medicines for millennia, but German chemists are responsible for so many of the current uses. In Europe, ginkgo biloba is a pharmaceutical herb. Ginkgo extract has been shown to be beneficial to the aged. This traditional plant boosts memory, focus, and other mental abilities by increasing oxygen usage. The plant compound has also been demonstrated to enhance long-distance eyesight and may even help to cure retinal degeneration. Its effectiveness in the management of depression in the elderly has also been shown in studies. People suffering from headaches, rhinitis, or dizziness may benefit from ginkgo extract. Tinnitus is a persistent buzzing in the ears that may be relieved with this supplement. It contains terpenoids and flavonoids, which increase blood flow and destroy microorganisms. Ginkgo Biloba is most often used to treat flu.

16. St. John's Wort

Hypericum, or St John's wort, is a medicinal herb. It's made from the leaves and flowers of the Hypericum perforatum plant, and it is often used as an herbal remedy for tissue

regeneration and psychological issues for generations. It is still widely available over-the-counter at health stores and pharmacies as depression therapy. However, since it includes biologically active substances, such as hypericin, it must be treated as a medicine. Although the underlying mechanism is disputed, it is thought to block norepinephrine and serotonergic reuptake, block MAO, increase the activity of serotonin receptors, and reduce serotonin receptor expression. Hepatitis B and herpes are the most common conditions for which St John's Wort is prescribed.

17. Oregano

Oregano is a fantastic plant to be used in your cuisine as well as for medicinal purposes. Oregano was venerated as a sign of bliss by the medieval Romans and Greeks, and the words mean "mountain joy." This is why paintings often represent newlyweds and grooms wearing oregano laurel crowns, which was a common custom at the period. Although oregano is widely used in Italian cuisine, it is best known in the United States as a pizza seasoning. This is a disservice to oregano, which comprises important vitamins A, C, E, and K, and also fiber, folate, iron, magnesium, vitamin B6, calcium, and potassium. Furthermore, oregano is frequently referred to as "wild marjoram" in European countries, and it is linked to the plant sweet marjoram. It includes strong phytonutrients that have the potential to be beneficial to one's body. It contains terpenes and thymol, both of which are antiviral. As a result, oregano is mostly used to treat chest problems.

18. Peppermint

Peppermint (Mentha piperita), a famous flavor for bubblegum, mouthwash, and beverages, may also help with indigestion and calm stomach cramps. It is often used to treat various ailments, itchy skin, anxiety, major depression, nausea, diarrhea, period pain, and gas due to its relaxing and soothing effect. It's also included in chest massages, which are used to alleviate the signs of the cold or flu. Peppermint inhibits the growth of bacteria, fungi, and viruses in laboratory tests, indicating that it has antibiotic, antimicrobial, and antiviral

effects. Peppermint has been shown to help with heartburn and gastrointestinal problems in many investigations. Polyphenols are found in it, and they help to combat viral infections. Peppermint is most often used to treat shingles and other viral infections.

19. Coriander

Coriander is a tiny Apiaceae plant with hollow stems that belongs to the family Coriandum. Coriandum sativum is its official nomenclature. The seeds have been used in food and as a component in different traditional treatments since olden history. They are pleasant, fragrant, and spicy. Coriander is a Mediterranean herb that is widely grown in Europe, the Mideast, Asia, India, and Turkey. In the west, it's known as cilantro. This annual plant with growing stems reaches up to 2 feet tall and has deep green velvety, hairless bi or tri-lobed leaflets. Tiny light pink blooms appear on the adult plant, which develops into spherical or oval-shaped fruits (seeds). The seeds are 4-6 millimeters in diameter and have an empty central chamber that contains medicinal essential oils. Monoterpenes are found in it, and they attack virus cells. Coriander is most often used to treat the common cold.

20. Oregon Grape Root

Acute and long-term urinary infections, skin problems like psoriasis and eczema, pimples, and painful blisters may all benefit from the Oregon grape. Pick the roots and stalks after the fruits have fallen down but before the new leaves grow from September to spring. This guarantees that the plant's essence, or health, is contained under the surface of the soil. The therapeutic skin on the branches and roots may be picked off and used raw in potions or dried for subsequent treatments. It contains isoquinoline alkaloids berberine and hydrasine. The cytomegalovirus, human papillomavirus, and herpes virus are all treated with Oregon Grape Root. It's available as a balm or as a pill. Just take 1–2 tablespoons of roughly sliced root and simmer for 10 minutes to make it into a drink. You may use it for no more than a week at a time, with at minimum a seven-day interval in between.

21. Ginger

Ginger has been used as a stomach medicine in China for at least two millennia, while its heritage in Asian food dates back to at least five thousand years. It was formerly thought by European people to have come straight from the Story of Creation, and it was used to brew beer by the early American immigrants. Many healers still use ginger to cure gastrointestinal diseases, but it has also shown promise in relieving the flu virus, motion sickness, and inflammation. It contains flavonoids that preserve healthy cells and stop viruses from reproducing. Ginger is also often used to treat common colds and flu.

After reading this book, you will not only have a better understanding of Dr. Sebi's ideology and herbal medicine, but you will also have a better understanding of the mechanisms by which careful food choices and the use of the right herbal ingredients can significantly affect your well-being, healing your body, and inhibiting the growth of harmful diseases. Dr. Sebi based the alkaline protocol on foods and herbs that have a lot of medicinal benefits and are supported with evidence. These advantages are there at your disposal. Coming from traditional pharmaceutical drugs to Dr. Sebi's alkaline herbal medicine is indeed a commitment. Dr. Sebi recommends a variety of herbal drinks to help your body repair itself. When you notice yourself craving a certain drink, try substituting it with any of the teas or a cooled healthy fruit juice. Make sure you have all of the alkaline herbs in your kitchen. The variety of taste choices expands your dining alternatives. Try substituting parsley for dill, or use the herbs indicated to transform a savory meal into a sweeter one. The more pleasure you have in the kitchen, the more likely you are to stick to your decision to use herbs and plants as medicine and reap long-term health benefits. The establishment of these substitute behaviors will be critical to the long-term success of your new healthy lifestyle.It's crucial to remember that your schedule and health aims should be based on your specific health issues. Let your body acclimate to novel plants by giving these herbs enough time to heal you, preferably a minimum of several weeks. Expect a detox component to your new lifestyle, particularly initially, while your body flushes itself off of mucous, acidity, and toxins. If you don't progressively add healthy plants into your diet, your digestive system may be shocked. If you have a pre-existing chronic condition, talk to your doctor or healthcare professional about the best course of action before using herbal remedies. Still, once you've committed to healing and detoxifying your body, there's no need to hurry. Rather than making a drastic change, create little, long-term modifications in your everyday life that will be a familiar and comfortable aspect of your habits. Test out every one of the herb varieties accessible to you and see which one works best for your specific condition.

Finally, every meaningful lifestyle change requires self-discipline, and selecting Dr. Sebi's alkaline herbs over traditional medication requires just that. It's a chance to pause and think about yourself. You may have investigated herbal medicine to treat your health problems for a variety of reasons. Whatever your reason, know that you have chosen the right path to health and longevity and that taking responsibility for those decisions will dramatically enhance your life. All of this is not to imply that it will be effortless since change is difficult. Allow yourself to be calm. You've already made the tough first step; now, it's only a matter of taking another one. Vow to take the first step toward better health and well-being. You have nothing to lose.

BOOK8:
Who Is Dr. Sebi?

The core tenet of the alkaline diet supports the concept that when acidic, or you can say acid-forming, foods are completely replaced with alkaline-based ones, the human body changes into an incredibly healthy metabolic engine. This is a concept that, to someone without any prior knowledge, would first seem a bit hard to comprehend, yet scientists across the globe have shown it to be true. The positive aspects of this alkaline diet have been seen to the point where it may help fend against illnesses like cancer.

These discoveries have gradually propelled the alkaline diet into the consciousness of millions of people worldwide, and we hope that you will be the next to recognize its benefits.

The Alkaline-Ash Diet, often known as the Acid Ash Diet, is the name by which the alkaline diet is most well-known worldwide. So, if you come across such names, don't become disoriented. However, they will explicitly call the diet an "Alkaline Diet" in the book for convenience. The major goal of the alkaline diet, as previously said, is basically to reduce the number of foods that are generally considered to be "acidic" and to allow the dietician to create a meal plan that enables them to consume foods that have an alkaline flavor. They often include a lot of fruits and vegetables.

Dr. Sebi is a naturalist, pathologist, biochemist, and herbalist. He has researched herbs and personally observed them, bringing his methods to our contemporary society. Dr. ebi diet promotes intercellular cleaning and revitalizing all the body's cells.

You will discover all of Dr. Sebi's remedies and therapeutic techniques in this book, along with how they may lower your chance of developing chronic and metabolic disorders. In this book, we'll talk about how to avoid cancer, heart attacks, and STDs and how to treat them and find remedies. In the next chapter, the Importance of an alkaline diet will be briefly explored, as well as its advantages.

Who Is Dr. Sebi?

Dr. Sebi is a biochemist, pathologist, herbalist, and naturalist. He has studied and personally experienced plants throughout North America, Central, and South America, Africa, and the Caribbean. He has developed a unique system and techniques for treating the human body with herbs firmly founded in more than 30 years of practice.

Alfredo Bowman, who would later become Dr. Sebi, was born in Ilanga, Spanish Honduras, on November 26, 1933. Dr. Sebi is a self-taught individual. Sebi's early experiences playing, seeing the river and the trees, and receiving guidance from his grandmother gave him the foundation he needed to live a life that was true to reality. He saw his adored grandma, who was aware of the movement of life.

Sebi, a self-educated guy with obesity, diabetes, impotence, and asthma, immigrated to the U.S. After receiving unsuccessful treatments from conventional doctors and well-known western medicine, Sebi decided to become a herbalist in Mexico. He began creating plant-based cell nutrition formulas specifically geared toward intercellular regeneration and redevelopment of all the body's defense cells, obtaining amazing therapeutic outcomes for all of his diseases. Dr. Sebi committed 30 years of his life to developing a novel strategy that he could only learn via years of scientific practice. Motivated by his recovery journey and the knowledge he gained, he began trading the compounds with others, giving birth to Dr. Sebi's Cell Food.

The Quest for Alkalinity

Sebi's main hypothesis seems to have been that alkaline foods and herbs (pH > 7) are adequate to control our body's acidity and that maintaining this alkaline state protects us against the mucus buildup that leads to sickness. To keep blood pH between 7.35 and 7.45, sodium bicarbonate and carbonic acid molecules are essential. The pH of our blood shouldn't be altered much. Above that is sickness and death. The high school biology fact, however, did not stop Sebi from selling a variety of herbal preparations.

1.2 Sebi's African Bio-mineral Balance Compounds

Simply said, Sebi's Cell Food items are plants, algae, and seaweed (also regarded as African Bio-mineral Equilibrium compounds). A container of their Bromide Plus pills costs $30 and is advertised as containing bladderwrack and "Irish sea moss," a kind of red algae." However, the component list is followed by the following worrisome note: " Dr. Sebi created the original and unique formulations for Sebi, which may include substances not listed here." I'm not sure about you, but I'm not at ease thinking about swallowing pills with unidentified substances." There may be a connection between these components and allergies, intolerances, or drugs that may interact with them. A significant liability results from failing to understand what they are.

But have they ever seen these chemicals performing the claimed functions? To regulate high or low blood pressure, use Sebi's Herbal Tea Blood Pressure Balance. Its only listed component is Flor de Manita, also called Chiranthodendron, a flowering plant native to

southern Mexico and Guatemala. Measurement of its effect on blood pressure should be straightforward, even if it has been "used for decades" to assist the heart (a claim from history that may not imply evidence of efficacy). However, the only studies dr. Sebi could find on this flower focused on its antibacterial properties in Petri dishes and its antiproliferative abilities in rats and mice. You won't be able to see your blood pressure.

Many Sebi chemicals are advertised as "detoxification" remedies, but it should be clear by this point that our bodies don't need a regular detox. Our kidneys and liver are quite effective at purifying our blood. The toxins that we are told to be afraid of are still vague and never adequately articulated, and these hazy boogeymen have never been shown to have a significant impact on the detoxification options suggested to us.

The African gene has stronger electrical vibration than other genes. However, Sebi's opinions on health went beyond the usual foolishness and into the pseudoscience of ethnicity. African genes have a strong electric resonance, according to Sebi, who also claimed that his African Bio-mineral Equilibrium naturally "compliments the structure of the African genome" in a letter to Zimbabwe's ambassador to the United States in 2002. Genes are not striking a chord. DNA segments rather than tuning forks code for proteins. In contrast, there is no such thing as an African gene. Most of our genetic variances are found among, not within, geographical groupings, which is one of the most often observed findings in the study of genetic variance in humans.

Then you may be concerned if genetic ancestry tests ask you if your great-grandparents were from Tunisia or Ireland. In your genome, they look for single-letter alterations and compare your pattern to a reference population that claims to be from a certain place, albeit their accuracy has come under scrutiny. There is no such thing as an African or European gene to pinpoint your ancestry further, even though these point mutations are dispersed throughout your DNA. The idea that your demand for food is determined by the frequency at which your genes vibrate is just rubbish.

1.3 Opening our Eyes

Self-taught specialists who claim to have identified the only cause of every sickness and the cure for it are common in the media. True science, regrettably, is slow, convoluted, and presents the idea of a dynamic cosmos in which different diseases have different causes and treatments are ineffective and have negative consequences. Dr. Sebi affected Facebook groups and accounts despite having tens of thousands of admirers.

1.4 Importance of Alkaline Body on Body and Mind

An alkaline diet, often known as electric food, is devoid of foods that contain acid and enables the body to heal itself. They are generally confined in nature. They promote the growth of iron, copper, and many other vital vitamins and minerals, all of which are necessary for a strong and effective immune system.

1.5 Acid – the illness builder

These were some of the most prevalent diseases often induced by acidic surroundings or society.

Allergy

An atmosphere that is too acidic is favorable for pollutants. Acidification and oxygen shortage often go hand in hand; an oxygen-deficient environment is conducive to the growth of harmful diseases, including fungus, viruses, and bacteria. While some beneficial bacteria are still present, most are toxic metabolic byproducts, which may undermine immunity and provide persistent pressure. The body becomes very sensitive to poisons and nutrients in this situation. Pollen and other foreign objects cause it to react, resulting in watery eyes, a runny nose, tissue swelling, etc. The body's efforts to eliminate acidic and toxic wastes are all unpleasant and life-threatening. Large amounts of acidic by-products are often produced by immune responses and allergic reactions, which may create dangerous circumstances for anybody with allergies. A cycle that can only be broken by slightly alkalinizing the blood.

Bone injuries

According to research published in several medical publications, including the European Journal, metabolic acid-base imbalances are connected to bone injuries, including fractures. Dr. Leon Root claims in his book that even a little drop in body pH can cause a sharp increase in bone loss.

BOOK:10

DR SEBI CANCER SOLUTION, CURE DIABETES AND remedies for ANXIETY

Cancer

Perhaps cancer is caused by more than simply our surroundings and way of life today. WHO started disseminating a global study on cancer that keeps tabs on incidence, prevalence, and mortality rates? According to analysis, only 4% of malignancies are genetic or inherited; the remainder is preventable and linked to lifestyle factors, including diet and environment.

Humans are electrical creatures, as are other living things. In the body, normal cells have a discernible negative electric charge. In an acidic and oxygen-deficient environment, cells play a beneficial electromagnetic function. Since opposites are included in the

electromagnetic rule, healthy and normal cells and their acids attract and cling to healthy cells. This increases the likelihood that healthy cells may be harmed by acidic environments or by cell fermentation, which happens when there is insufficient oxygen.

If the amount of bad tissue increases in live, healthy cells, the body also produces a defense mechanism to separate and cover the tissue to stop it from spreading. The tumor is the term for this. Many holistic healthcare experts see cancer as a pervasive influence rather than an illness. These disparities act as metabolic stressors. Acids are transferred throughout cells, tissues, and organs as they build up in the blood.

Dr. Sebi & Cancer Cure

Although cancer is a basic problem, it is important to provide some facts. When some individuals learn about cancer treatments, they believe that after the disease has been eliminated from the body, they will no longer have cancer. This is a clear, sensible idea, yet it conflicts with the complexity of cancer.

Cancer develops when cells gradually depart from their environment of origin. Typically, this happens gradually over the years or even decades.

It does not mean that every divergence from the norm or normal circumstance is malignant. Through the ongoing process of cell regeneration, cells continuously diverge from their initial condition. Several things will happen as a result of this, including: o The Cell will reconstructing itself

- The Cell will commit suicide (apoptosis).

- The cell will be destroyed by the immunological reaction.

- The Cell does nothing except sit still, not growing or reproducing (senescence).

Therefore, the body experiences cell divergence and correction as a normal daily process.

Only when certain processes fail can cancer spread. We assert that cells become cancerous when they become "malignant." Malignancy often has two characteristics: cells infiltrate surrounding tissue, start to differentiate when they shouldn't, and spread (i.e., metastasis) to other parts of the body. Two distinguishing characteristics of cancer are unregulated cell growth and a propensity to spread throughout the body.

Therefore, when we talk about treating sickness, we mean preventing these two occurrences via natural means.

We can never forbid cells from deviating from the norm, and we may not even want to. Cell divergence has generated survival advantages over millions of years, allowing humans to evolve from inconspicuous, center-of-the-food-chain primates to become the dominant

species on the planet. In other words, Darwinian evolution is a result of advantageous cell differentiation.

Cancer is the negative separation byproduct or the opposite side of the coin.

Therefore, when we discuss a cure for cancer, we refer to removing the harmful effects of cells that deviate from their normal condition. In other words, there is no chance that cancer cells will reappear since they have all disappeared from the body.

Many naturalists have slightly varied opinions regarding how to treat cancer. If cancer can be treated for an extended period using natural and other medicines, they contend that cancer is basically "cured." Here, natural treatments stop it in its tracks so that the patient may live a normal life. This paradigm is used for other diseases where treatment might take decades due to improvements in medical science, such as HIV.

6.1 Latest Chemotherapy Methods

Chemotherapy is a synthetic poison that ill people and has very dangerous side effects.

Cancer cells seem to develop swiftly, while chemotherapy drugs kill quickly growing cells. However, since these drugs go throughout the body, they will also affect healthy, natural cells capable of rapid growth. Chemotherapy harms both healthy and normal cells, and the bone marrow's blood-forming cells are the normal cells most likely to be harmed by chemotherapy.

- Reproductive system cells,
- the mouth and the digestive tract.
- Follicles for hair.

The heart, kidney, gut, lungs, and nerve cells may all be destroyed by chemotherapy medicines.

6.2 Cancer Cure Through Natural Ways

The body is a wonderful, dynamic system designed to self-correct. It was designed to fend against and defeat the illness, heal weakening cells, and, when necessary, obliterate severely damaged cells. The body consistently functions throughout a person's life cycle by replacing worn-out cells with new ones via cell replication. This is how the body maintains the overall health of the tissues and blood. Most body cells replace themselves and eventually die in a process called apoptosis. On average, red blood cells change every four months, bones every ten years, the digestive tract and lining every five days, and the skin every two to four weeks. It was formerly thought that brain cells could not be repaired; however, current research is reevaluating this idea. Proteins and hormones are used by the body to carry out various functions.

Phytonutrients assist such molecules in maintaining the defense of their growing organs. This nature is so complex that an intelligent order could have only created it. People's bodies may utilize chemical compounds to strengthen their immune systems when they consume phytonutrients from plants. These phytonutrients may help regenerate DNA, detoxify, and attach pollutants so they can be removed from the body, enhance cell communication, get rid of germs, and function as antioxidants to protect cells from free radical damage and aging. They may also help kill cancer cells. Various phytonutrients interact with the body differently, such as flavonoids, carotenoids, isothiocyanates, phytates, indoles, phenols, saponins, sulfides, and terpenes.

BOOK 11:

CURE DIABETES AND remedies

for ANXIETY

Anxiety

Suicidal symptoms might resemble those of an acidic body or one with a microbial overgrowth. Acid-forming substances include tobacco, illicit drugs, dangerous chemicals, and other organic compounds. Trans fats, food coloring and additives, organic packaging, prescription medications, and carbs started to be utilized for depression.

Diabetes

Diabetes still exists in many forms. Due to the pancreas' inability to create any insulin on its own, type 1 diabetes is insulin dependent. The individual becomes to rely on external sources of insulin, including insulin injections, for the rest of their lives.

Poor eating habits and an insufficient amount of insulin stored in the pancreas seem to be the causes of type 2 diabetes. Consequently, the body's ability to use insulin to do this is diminished. It is crucial for people with diabetes to maintain blood sugar levels within a certain range at all times and to avoid the substantial spikes in blood sugar brought on by eating sweets.

In addition to producing insulin, which helps regulate blood sugar levels by transferring blood sugar to cells for energy, the pancreas also produces alkaline fluid for the body. There are digestive enzymes in the fluid. Mold, yeast, and fungal growth in an acidic environment might affect the pancreas' function and the body's ability to digest sugar.

1.6 Body pH and Importance

Why is pH balance so important? Perhaps you know how important pH is for keeping a pool or growing plants. pH balance in people is also essential to the body. The pH of many bodily parts varies, but we'll focus on the pH of the blood component.

Similar to body temperature, blood acid/alkaline balance can only move or fluctuate within a very small, tightly controlled range. The blood's pH, which is 7.365, is somewhat alkaline. The body is constantly undergoing precise modifications to keep it in the proper position. These changes can be connected. To maintain homeostasis, we shiver to warm up or sweat to cool down. Like food, emotions, and environmental contaminants, the majority tend to alter the blood's pH, which may cause them to respond. It is difficult for the blood to become overly alkaline due to the enormous numbers and variety of acids to which we are accustomed. The body uses a variety of clever acid removal strategies to maintain a properly maintained pH. Ironically, those with very alkaline blood have too acidic bodies; in this case, the blood releases alkaline particles to balance it.

Multiple processes are still in progress to prevent the chronic and ongoing effects of the acids we are exposed to via food, our environment, and our metabolism (producing and consuming energy creates acid).

Organs are involved in eliminating toxic compounds via the intestines, urine, sweat, and sometimes acidic exhale through gas respiration (CO_2).

Baking soda, or sodium bicarbonate, is also produced by the body to balance and neutralize acidity. Due to the inherent salinity of our blood, salt is utilized to treat it. Bicarbonate sodium is a key component of our defense against acids. Omega 3 and omega 6 oils may be used by the body to balance the acidity.

As a result, we should eat a variety of meals that are balanced and rich in alkaline minerals and good fats. When we sometimes get excessively acidic, our body removes some waste and draws the necessary alkaline deposits.

Strategies to Surpass Diabete

It suggests that if you had diabetes, your blood glucose, also known as blood sugar, would be excessively high. Insulin, a hormone, is often utilized to aid in converting food into energy. When someone develops diabetes, their body is either unable to produce insulin or uses it improperly. If diabetes is not controlled, it may result in serious health issues, renal failure, heart disease, and blindness. Diabetes may be managed by eating a balanced diet, exercising more, and keeping blood sugar levels within an acceptable range. You must elevate the eating experience. As it is often known, type ll diabetes is mostly a lifestyle disease that may be controlled by changing one's diet. An alkaline diet based on plants is safer. Because mucus is the root of all illnesses, according to Dr. Sebi, the body is more prone to be in an acidic state. Where the disease is present, mucus would be prevalent. Dr. Sebi assisted millions of individuals with diabetes via his approach, and his passing did not affect this. He also left behind treatment techniques for diabetes. Here is a detailed analysis of Dr. Sebi's diabetic treatment, and you will get insight from his attitude on how seriously he took this deadly disease.

7.1 Natural remedies for type 2 diabetes

Diabetes type 2 (also known as diabetes mellitus) results from a cascade of factors, including insufficient exercise, eating too many unhealthy foods, being stressed out, having insomnia, consuming toxins, and heredity. Patients with type 2 diabetes commonly use natural remedies and conventional therapy to address their disease. Using natural cures and pharmaceuticals is a great approach to augmenting your diabetes care. However, if used without the right knowledge or guidelines, mixing herbs, nutrients, and pharmaceuticals might result in hypoglycemia and a drop in blood sugar levels.

The following is a list of all-natural remedies for type 2 diabetes.

Apple cider vinegar

The primary component of ACV, acetic acid, is thought to be responsible for some of its health benefits. There are several evidence-based ways to use ACV. Two tablespoons taken before night might reduce your blood sugar levels. Even better, adding 1-2 tablespoons of ACV to meals helps lower the glycemic index of a meal that is high in carbs. Patients are instructed to consume ACV either on its own or combined with teas and salad dressings before a meal.

Barley and fiber

Consuming fiber lowers insulin and blood sugar levels. The recommended daily fiber intake is about 30 grams, and most Americans only consume 6 to 8 grams, which is insufficient. Although you could think about using fiber supplements like Metamucil, eating your vegetables is the best way to reach your goal! A high-protein, high-fiber grain like barley has been shown to reduce inflammation overall and increase levels of insulin, cholesterol, and blood sugar. Barley often cooks on the stovetop in less than fifteen minutes with only a little water and salt, and it does not need soaking.

Chromium

Brewer's yeast contains most of the chromium; chromium shortage affects glucose metabolism. Facts back up the use of chromium for decreased A1c and blood sugar levels. But if you have renal problems, use caution while using this supplement.

Zinc

Zinc deficiency is often detected in people with diabetes. Studies on the effects of zinc supplementation have shown that it may decrease A1C and blood sugar, have antioxidant activity, lower blood sugar levels, and even assist manage issues associated with diabetes. You should be prepared to call for the proper dosage recommendations since high quantities of zinc will inhibit the absorption of other minerals, such as copper.

Aloe vera

The sap of the aloe vera plant is well known for its laxative properties. So be sure to drink the gel juice! There is mounting evidence that gel—the mucilaginous component found within the leaves—is being employed. To avoid needing to use the restroom, make sure any product you purchase is anthraquinone- or aloin-free!

Berberine

Existing studies support that it is used to lower blood sugar and hba1c levels. Due to potential interactions with the metabolism of conventional pharmaceuticals, this plant should never be used while pregnant.

Cinnamon

Cinnamon is safe for medicinal use and lowers cholesterol and blood sugar levels.

Fenugreek

Fenugreek lowers hba1c and cholesterol levels. This plant may sometimes cause one's urine to smell like maple syrup, although this is not hazardous.

Gymnema

Evidence supporting benefits for glucose metabolism as an alternative to enhancing insulin levels and traditional medicines is beginning to catch up with its clinical usage.

Nopal

Reduce the amount of sugar in your blood.

7.2 Herbal and Natural Therapies

Many popular spices and herbs are said to have blood sugar-lowering effects, making them beneficial for those who have type 2 diabetes or are at high risk of developing it.

The usage of these more "natural" components by people with diabetes to manage their illness has increased in recent years due to various medical studies that suggest potential connections between herbal medicines and improved blood glucose control.

What are natural remedies available?

Certain plants are anti-diabetic. What follows is a list of some of those plants: Cinnamon, fenugreek, aloe vera, bilberry extract, okra, ginger, bitter melon

Further herbal therapies

Native Americans have traditionally employed the plants and herb derivatives listed below to treat diabetes in the regions where they thrive.

Allium sativum

Allium sativum, often known as garlic, is hypothesized to provide antioxidant and micro-circulatory effects. Despite the limited number of research that has directly connected allium to insulin and blood glucose levels, the outcomes have been promising. Allium may boost secretion, lower blood sugar levels, and decrease insulin deterioration.

Coccinia indica

The 'ivy gourd,' also known as Coccinia indica, is planted extensively over the Indian subcontinent. The plant, which has long been utilized in ayurvedic medicine, was shown to contain characteristics that mimic insulin (i.e., it imitates the insulin function).

Ficus carica

Although the active element in fig-leaf, or Ficus Carican, is unclear, it is widely recognized in Spain and South-West Europe as a diabetic remedy. According to several animal studies, the fig leaf promotes glucose absorption.

Ginseng

The name "ginseng" refers to several different plant species. Some research utilizing American ginseng showed a reduction in fasting blood glucose. Ginseng from Siberia, America, Japan, Korea, and other regions are among the varieties. In certain locations, the plant, particularly the Panax species, is revered as a "cure-all." More extensive research is needed to confirm ginseng's effectiveness, as is the case for many herbs used to treat diabetes across the globe.

Gymnema Sylvestre

Additionally used in Ayurvedic herbal treatment is gymnema silvestre. The plant, which thrives in the tropical woods of Southern and Central India, has been associated with a considerable reduction in blood sugar levels. According to certain animal studies, there has been an improvement in beta-cell activity and islet cell regeneration.

Momordica charantia

Momordica Some parts of Africa, South America, and Asia are home to the charantia plant. This is sold as charantia, but it's also referred to as bitter melon, karolla, or karela. The plant may be prepared in several ways, helping those with diabetes produce insulin and oxidize glucose, among other things. Their immediate impact on blood sugar levels is also notable.

Ocimum sanctum

Ocimum sanctum, sometimes known as holy basil, is a plant used in traditional medicine. A controlled clinical experiment showed a favorable effect on postprandial and fasting glucose levels, and experts anticipate that the herb may enhance beta cell activity and encourage insulin release.

Opuntia streptacantha

Opuntia streptacantha, sometimes known as the prickly-pear cactus, is a common plant in the dry regions where it breeds.

The plant in charge of glucose has traditionally been used by those living in the Mexican desert. Animal studies have demonstrated significant reductions in HbA1c, postprandial glucose, and HbA1c, and certain plant characteristics may impact intestinal absorption of glucose.

Again, more clinical studies are necessary to prove the effectiveness of the prickly-pear cactus as a treatment for diabetes patients.

Silybum marianum

As a member of the aster family, Silybum marianum is often known as milk thistle. High amounts of flavonoids and antioxidants are produced by silymarin, and both may help reduce insulin resistance. The effect of Silybum marianum in glycemic regulation is poorly understood.

Some herbs are also being researched, and they could benefit diabetes people. Following is a list of some of them:

Curry, Cinnamomum tamala, Pterocarpus marsupium, Eugenia jambolana, Gingko, Phyllanthus amarus, Solanum torvum, Vinca rosea, and others

The Dr. Sebi diet encourages consuming uncooked, natural meals from plants. It may help you lose weight, but it's quite restricted, deficient in certain nutrients, mainly depends on taking the creator's pricey supplements, and falsely claims to turn your body into an alkaline condition. Many alternative healthy diets are more adaptable and durable if you want to adopt a more plant-based eating pattern. Scientific studies do not support the Dr. Sebi diet. It could, however, provide certain advantages like other plant-based diets. Increased consumption of entire fruits and vegetables may improve health, and if losing weight is a goal, it could also aid in that.

The Dr. Sebi diet's limitations, however, could be dangerous. When required, it is critical to ensure the body gets adequate nutrients, especially vitamin B-12. The dangers of the Dr. Sebi diet may affect certain individuals more than others. Adolescents, nursing mothers, and elderly folks are among them. No scientific research supports the use of the goods that the diet's proponents advise. Eating more plant-based meals and taking supplements for any lacking nutrients could be a more beneficial strategy. Before attempting any new diet, it may be a good idea to do some research and speak with a healthcare provider.

Whatever path you choose, it's important to create a perception of balance in your life. An alkaline diet is increasingly crucial because acidic elements govern our lifestyle. The commoners' immune systems have been further weakened by excessive chemical medication use, making them more susceptible to the complicated illnesses of today's world.

BOOK 12:

Dr. Sebi's Diet

This diet was developed by herbalist Alfredo Darrington Bowman, often known as Dr. Sebi, and is based on the African Bio-Mineral Balance philosophy. Despite his name, Dr. Sebi was neither a medical doctor nor a Ph.D.

He created this diet for anybody who wants to enhance their general health, organically treat or prevent illness, and avoid using traditional Western medicine.

Dr. Sebi claims that every part of your body where mucus builds up might lead to sickness. He said that diabetes is brought on by an abundance of mucus in the pancreas, while pneumonia is brought on by a buildup of mucus in the lungs.

He suggested that illnesses start when your body gets too acidic and cannot thrive in an alkaline environment. His diet and expensive, proprietary supplements promise to cleanse your sick body and return it to its original alkaline condition.

Initially, Dr. Sebi said that this diet could treat diseases including lupus, leukemia, sickle cell disease, and AIDS. However, he was told to stop making them follow a 1993 lawsuit.

The diet consists of a certain set of permitted grains, nuts, seeds, fruits, vegetables, oils, and herbs. The Dr. Sebi diet is considered vegan since animal products are not allowed.

According to Sebi, you must adhere to the diet religiously for the rest of your life if you want your body to repair itself.

Finally, despite the claims of many that the program has cured them, no scientific studies back up these assertions.

2.1 How to Follow the Dr. Sebi Diet?

The Dr. Sebi diet has extremely rigorous guidelines. These are included on his website:

Rule 1: Stick to the foods recommended in the nutritional guide.

Rule 2: Every day, consume one gallon (3.8 liters) of water.

Rule 3: Consume Dr. Sebi's vitamins one hour before taking medicine.

Rule 4: No animal products are allowed.

Rule 5: No alcohol is permitted.

Rule 6: Eat only the "natural-growing grains" in the manual and avoid wheat products.

Rule 7: To avoid "killing" your food, don't use the microwave.

Rule 8: Stay away from canned or seedless fruit.

There are no recommendations for nutrients. However, since it forbids beans, lentils, pork, and soy products, this diet is poor in protein. Essential food for healthy muscles, skin, and joints is protein.

Additionally, you are required to buy Dr. Sebi's "cell food" supplements, which claim to cleanse and replenish your body's cells.

There are no suggestions for particular supplements. You are required to place a purchase for any supplement that addresses your health issues instead.

For instance, the "Bio Ferro" capsules make the following claims: they heal liver problems, purify the blood, strengthen immunity, encourage weight reduction, help digestive problems, and improve general wellbeing.

It's difficult to determine whether the supplements will satisfy your daily requirements since they don't provide a comprehensive list of nutrients or their dosages.

2.2 Dr. Sebi Diet Vs. A Vegan Diet

It's reasonable to assume that this is merely another vegan diet in a different package, given the abundance of plant-based items on Dr. Sebi's recommended food list. A vegan diet, however, allows soy products and many kinds of beans and legumes, but none of these are allowed on the Dr. Sebi food list. This is one of the main distinctions between the Dr. Sebi diet and a vegan diet. Anybody who follows the Dr. Sebi diet for an extended period would find it very challenging to consume enough protein due to eliminating beans and legumes. Additionally, the Dr. Sebi diet limits fruits and vegetables that it deems to be overly acidic, in contrast to standard vegan diets that include any fruit or vegetable. Thus, according to Amanda Kostro Miller, RD, LDN, most individuals are likely to find this diet much too restricted.

2.3 Can the Dr. Sebi Diet Help You Lose Weight?

Even though Dr. Sebi's diet isn't intended to help you lose weight, doing so is possible if you stick to it.

A Western diet that is heavy in ultra-processed foods and packed with salt, sugar, fat, and calories are discouraged by the diet.

Instead, it encourages eating whole, plant-based foods. Plant-based diets encourage lower rates of obesity and heart disease compared to the Western diet.

In 12-month research involving 65 participants, it was shown that individuals who consumed an unrestricted amount of whole foods and low-fat plant-based meals shed more pounds than those who did not.

At six months, the diet group had dropped an average of 26.6 pounds (12.1 kg), whereas the control group had lost just 3.5 pounds (1.6 kg).

Aside from nuts, seeds, avocados, and oils, most of the items on this diet are low in calories. Therefore, it's doubtful that eating a lot of things that are allowed will cause you to consume too many calories and gain weight.

Extremely low-calorie diets, however, are often impossible to follow over the long term. Most dieters who use these plans gain the weight back after returning to regular eating habits.

It's impossible to determine if this diet will give adequate calories for long-term weight reduction since it doesn't include instructions for amounts and portions.

2.4 Potential Benefits of the Dr. Sebi Diet

The Dr. Sebi diet's heavy focus on plant-based meals is one of its advantages.

The diet emphasizes eating a lot of fruits and vegetables since they are rich in fiber, vitamins, minerals, and plant-based substances. Diets high in fruits and vegetables have been linked to lowered oxidative stress and inflammation and protection against various illnesses.

According to research including 65,226 adults, those who had seven or more servings of fruit and vegetables each day had a 25% and 31% reduced incidence of heart disease and cancer, respectively.

Additionally, the majority of individuals consume too little fresh vegetables. According to one study, just 9.3% and 12.2% of Americans consumed the recommended amounts of fruit and vegetables.

Additionally, the Dr. Sebi diet encourages the use of whole grains high in fiber and healthy fats, including nuts, seeds, and plant oils. A decreased risk of heart disease has been associated with some foods.

Finally, diets that exclude items that have undergone extreme processing are linked to improved diet quality overall.

Among the potential health advantages of a plant-based diet are:

- Weight loss: According to 2015 research, a vegan diet led to more weight reduction than other, less limiting diets. After six months on a vegan diet, participants had dropped up to 7.5 percent of their body weight.

- Controlling appetite – A 2016 research of young male participants discovered that they felt more content and fuller after consuming a plant-based meal that included peas and beans as opposed to a meal that included meat.

- Modifying the microbiome—the bacteria in the gut are collectively referred to as the "microbiome." A plant-based diet may modify the microbiome positively, lowering the risk of illness, according to 2016 research. More investigation will be needed to verify this, however.

- Lower risk of illness – A 2017 research found that a plant-based diet may cut the chance of developing metabolic syndrome and type 2 diabetes in half, as well as the risk of coronary heart disease by 40%.

2.5 Downsides of the Dr. Sebi Diet

Remember that this diet has several disadvantages.

Highly Restrictive

Dr. Sebi's diet prohibits a wide variety of foods, including all animal products, lentils, wheat, beans, and several kinds of vegetables and fruits, which is a significant drawback.

It is so rigorous that just a few kinds of fruit are permitted. For instance, beefsteak or Roma tomatoes are not permitted; only cherry or plum tomatoes are.

Furthermore, a rigorous diet may not be pleasurable to follow. It may result in a bad connection with food, particularly given that it denigrates items that aren't included in its nutrition guide.

Finally, this diet promotes additional bad habits like using supplements to feel full. Since supplements don't provide many calories, this assertion encourages unhealthful eating habits.

Lacks Protein and other Essential Nutrients

The foods Dr. Sebi recommends in his nutrition advice may be a fantastic source of nutrients.

Protein, a necessary component for skin structure, muscular development, and the manufacturing of hormones and enzymes, isn't included in any of the approved meals, however.

Only a few nuts—walnuts, sesame seeds, Brazil nuts, and hemp seeds—are allowed, and even those aren't very high in protein. For instance, 4 and 9 grams of protein are present in 1/4 cup (25 grams) of walnuts and 3 tablespoons (30 grams) of hemp seeds, respectively.

You would need to consume unusually big servings of these items to achieve your daily protein requirements.

Although the foods in this diet are rich in certain nutrients like beta carotene, potassium, and the vitamins C and E, they are deficient in other elements like omega-3, calcium, iron, and the vitamins D and B12, which are frequent nutrients to worry about for those who follow a strictly plant-based diet.

According to the Dr. Sebi diet website, some of the supplements' constituents are proprietary. This is worrisome since it's impossible to determine if you'll achieve your daily

nutritional requirements because it's unknown which nutrients you're receiving and in what amounts.

Not Based on Science

The absence of scientific backing for Dr. Sebi's nutrition strategy is one of the greatest issues.

The diet claims that its meals and supplements regulate your body's creation of acids. Although it naturally makes your body somewhat alkaline, the human body rigorously controls its acid-base balance to preserve blood pH values between 7.36 and 7.44.

Rare circumstances, such as diabetic ketoacidosis, might cause blood pH to deviate from this range. Without quick medical care, this might be lethal.

Finally, research has revealed that nutrition may briefly and modestly alter the pH of your urine but not your blood. Thus, according to Dr. Sebi, the diet won't result in your body being more alkaline.

2.6 Is the Dr. Sebi diet Safe?

Dr. Sebi's diet is quite limited and leaves out several necessary elements. This diet may allow your body to survive for a little period, but it isn't long-term sustainable or healthful. Additionally, no diet may make your blood more alkaline.

As this diet excludes foods high in protein, omega-3 fatty acids, calcium, iron, vitamin D, and vitamin B12, following it for more than a few weeks may leave you susceptible to micronutrient shortages and malnutrition.

Those with osteoporosis, osteopenia, or iron deficiency anemia may have particular difficulties from these lacking minerals. Since it is deficient in essential micronutrients, the Dr. Sebi diet may make these illnesses worse.

Pernicious anemia, which may cause exhaustion, memory issues, shortness of breath, a pins-and-needles sensation in your hands and feet, and a raw, red tongue, can also result from a lack of vitamin B12.

This diet is dangerous for certain populations, including individuals with a history of or current eating disorders and pregnant women.

Before starting this diet, those with renal illness should speak with a doctor or qualified dietitian.

2.7 Are Alkaline Foods Healthier?

The concepts of "alkaline meals" and "detoxifying rituals" are not accepted in modern medicine. Suppose individuals maintain a balanced diet, engage in regular physical activity, and consume foods high in antioxidants, polyphenols, and fiber. In that case, their bodies will continue to detoxify themselves as long as their liver and kidneys are in good condition.

Numerous studies have shown that an alkaline diet has no advantages. Instead, such diets may result in serious nutritional deficits, such as a lack of protein (Dr. Sebi's diet is particularly low in protein), iron deficiency anemia, vitamin B12 insufficiency, and vitamin B12 deficiency.

Dr. Sebi's alkaline diet has the benefits of being rich in fiber and whole foods and reducing caffeine and nicotine use. If adhered to diligently, it could lead to weight reduction. The high fiber content improves intestinal flora, regulates blood sugar levels, and stops binge eating.

There is no proof that an alkaline diet prevents malignancies or autoimmune diseases, despite being high in fiber and low in sugar. The plants used in the cleaning process may negatively react to people's medications.

In large dosages, several of the alkaline "herbs" may be hazardous to the body. It is essential to go through any drastic dietary changes with your doctor.

2.8 Foods to Eat on the Dr. Sebi Diet

The restricted list of foods in Dr. Sebi's nutrition manual includes:

Fruits: apples, cantaloupe, papayas, currants, figs, elderberries, dates, berries, peaches, seeded key limes, prickly pears, soft jelly coconuts, seeded melons, mangoes, Latin or West Indies soursop, and tamarind.

Brazil nuts, raw sesame seeds, raw tahini butter, hemp seeds, and walnuts are among the nuts and seeds. Among the oils are avocado oil, unrefined coconut oil, grapeseed oil, hemp seed oil, unrefined olive oil, and sesame oil.

Spices include oregano, bay leaf, habanero, tarragon, basil, cloves, onion powder, dill, sweet basil, achiote, cayenne, sage, pure agave syrup, powdered, granulated seaweed, and date sugar. Herbal teas include elderberry, tila, burdock, chamomile, fennel, ginger, and raspberry.

You may also swig water along with the tea.

Additionally, you are allowed to consume grains in the pasta, bread, cereal, or flour. However, any meal that uses yeast or baking soda to leaven it is forbidden.

2.9 Which Foods Are Alkaline Rich?

There is no scientific justification for restricting your diet to solely the items mentioned above since your diet has no appreciable impact on the pH of your blood.

The majority of fruits, vegetables, nuts, and whole grains are foods that promote alkalinity. According to research, eating a mix of these foods increases lifespan and improves health.

Therefore, there are several benefits to increasing your intake of plant-based meals. In other words, meals that are good for your health go beyond the items on Dr. Sebi's list.

As a result, you need to think about including these items in a balanced diet:

- Fresh coconut, bananas, and kiwis are among the fruits. Among the vegetables are potatoes, Swiss chard, broccoli, Brussels sprouts, iceberg lettuce, cauliflower, and soybeans.

- Beans and lentils are legumes.

- Proteins: tofu

2.10 Foods to Avoid on The Dr. Sebi Diet

Foods like are prohibited if they aren't included in Dr. Sebi's nutrition guide.

- Eggs, dairy, dairy products, fish, red meat, chicken, canned fruit and vegetables, seedless fruit, poultry, and soy products.

- Fortified meals, such as those from restaurants or take-out services.

- Other than date sugar and agave syrup, wheat, sugar, and alcohol

- foods produced with baking powder; or yeast or foods raised with yeast.

Numerous cereals, fruits, vegetables, nuts, and seeds are prohibited.

2.11 Sample Menu and Recipes

Here is an example meal for the Dr. Sebi diet for three days.

Day 1	Day 2	Day 3
Breakfast: 2 banana-spelled pancakes with agave syrup	Breakfast: shake made with hemp seeds, water, strawberries, and bananas	Breakfast: cooked quinoa with agave syrup, pure coconut milk, and peaches
Lunch: Kale salad with tomatoes, dandelion greens, onions, chickpeas, and avocados	Lunch: homemade pizza, using a spelt flour crust, vegetables, and Brazil nut cheese	Lunch: spelt pasta with chopped vegetables with olive oil and key lime dressing
Dinner: Vegetable and wild rice stir fry	Dinner: chickpea burger with kale, onion, tomato, on spelt flour flatbread	Dinner: vegetable soup using red peppers, onions, water, spices, kale, mushrooms

BOOK 13:

Dr. Sebi's Treatment

Dr. Sebi, a Honduran-born scientist, pathologist, and herbalist, was Alfredo Darrington Bowman, better known by his stage name Dr. Sebi. He was born into extremely modest circumstances. He worked for over three decades to find treatments for various illnesses, including cancer, epilepsy, diabetes, herpes, gonorrhea, HIV, AIDS, syphilis, and lupus. Along with other sexually transmitted illnesses, he also developed the Dr. Sebi treatment for herpes and AIDS.

3.1 Healing with "Electric" & Botanical Foods

Eliminating excessive mucus, which Dr. Sebi thought to be the cause of all sickness, is the basis of his therapeutic approach. He added that having too much mucus causes bronchitis, diabetes, pneumonia, and arthritis when it accumulates in the lungs, pancreatic duct, or joints.

3.2 Why Is There So Much Mucus?

According to Dr. Sebi, food is the primary cause of the body's mucus overproduction. One of the culprits is starch, a substance that harms health since it increases body acidity. Animal products work similarly, and an acidic body will produce poisonous mucus, clog the system and create inflammation.

Dr. Sebi Alkaline Foods List:

Dr. Sebi advised fasting in addition to the correct food to cleanse every cell and replenish mineral deficiencies. Dr. Sebi divided food into six categories: raw, living, hybrid, dead, genetically modified, and pharmaceuticals. His healing diet encouraged individuals to eat a mostly raw vegan diet by eliminating all food types except live and raw. These raw foods are now often referred to as "living" foods. According to Dr. Sebi, live foods are "electric," which means they can combat the body's acidic food waste.

3.3 Suppression of Dr. Sebi Herpes Cure

The theories of Dr. Sebi are in opposition to U.S. traditional medicine. It is true that the medical industry continues to look for and advocate for novel treatments for several illnesses, including COVID, diabetes, Alzheimer's, and cancer. The medical establishment, however, sees Dr. Sebi's strategy as a danger and manages to disprove it. For instance, the Dr. Sebi treatment for cancer and other Dr. Sebi cures, including the Dr. Sebi herpes cure, challenge long-standing therapy regimens.

However, organ replacement technology represents one of the fascinating recent advancements in medicine and offers a peek at the future of human anatomy. Here are a few instances:

- A paradigm for an artificial kidney was successfully tested, bringing hope to relieve renal disease patients off transplant lists and dialysis equipment.

- After receiving the first artificial cornea, a man regains his vision.

In this regard, it should be noted that Dr. Sebi would surely assert that his treatment for renal illness would remove the need for dialysis.

BOOK 14:

Dr. Sebi Cure for Herpes and Other Sexually Transmitted Diseases (STDs)

Dr. Sebi's therapies for STDs were one of his areas of expertise. STDs are illnesses readily transmitted from person to person, result in several difficulties, and are sometimes hard to treat with traditional medication. STDs are often linked and may be brought on by bacteria, fungi, parasites, and viruses. Some of them make other sexually transmitted illnesses more likely to develop and have symptoms that make them difficult to differentiate.

3.5 How Can STDs Be Prevented?

It is possible to transmit STDs, venereal illnesses, and many forms of sexual activity (oral, genital, and anal). The body's immune system determines a person's sensitivity to this form

of disease and infection. Therefore the less efficient the immune system is, the greater the likelihood that a person would have a sexually transmitted virus (STIs).

One of the most frequent pathogenic origins of STDs is bacteria, followed by viruses and parasites. According to a phytochemical study, plant products are a great source of phenols, antioxidants, and physiologically active chemicals. They are also essential for several bacterial and viral illnesses and STDs and may have a deterrent effect on germs and infectious viruses. According to Dr. Sebi, this chapter references some of the most important therapeutic herbs that have inhibitory effects on the spread and multiplication of pathogenic organisms linked to STDs.

There is evidence that several plants may prevent and cure genital tract illnesses and STDs and serve as antibacterial and antiviral agents.

Through phytochemical research, medicinal plants' therapeutic and clinical advantages have been investigated, and how to use their active components to create herbal medications has been addressed. These plants may be utilized to produce herbal medications that reduce genital tract infections (microbial, bacterial, and fungal), STDs, and pain in patients due to their vital flavonoids and active ingredients.

Everybody may take precautions to lessen their risk of developing an STD. The fundamental advice is to practice safe monogamy, use condoms if you have any doubts about your relationship, and contact your doctor regularly for checkups. Regular STD screenings are also advised.

3.6 Herbal treatment for STDs and genital tract infections

Apple vinegar

In addition to being a very powerful cleaner and antibiotic, apple vinegar also has antifungal and antibacterial properties that enhance the body's immunological response to harmful organisms.

Rosemary

Several infectious disorders are treated using rosemary, a plant with antibacterial and anti-inflammatory properties. Utilizing the tea or oily extract of the plant is the finest technique to alter the qualities of rosemary.

Garlic

Garlic is a powerful natural antibiotic with a microbicidal antibacterial action and is highly effective in treating various illnesses. The extract of this plant lessens pain and prevents vaginal yeast illnesses.

Tea tree oil

With its strong antibiotic, antifungal, and antibacterial properties, tea tree oil effectively treats infection to treat gynecological diseases.

Basil leaf

The active microbicide in basil leaves may suppress various bacteria and fungus.

Aloe vera

Application of Aloe vera, using A. Vera and its gel are helpful in illness prevention and contribute to itching relief. The nectar of the plant reduces infection-related irritation in the genitals.

Blueberries

Fruits like blueberries are suggested to avoid disorders of the urinary system and have several uses in traditional therapies. The bacterium that causes the illness in the body and prevents its proliferation and accumulation may be eliminated by a chemical substance in the fruit known as PACS. Consuming blueberries is effective in getting rid of fungal diseases.

Oak

The leaves and bark of an oak tree include oil, pectin, mucilage, tannin, quercetin, resin,

sugar, malic acid, and gallic acid. Consequently, this plant has a very high capability for killing germs, which significantly reduces the risk of infectious illness and STDs in the genital tract and helps treat them.

Eucalyptus

Eucalyptus essential oil has antibacterial properties that are effective against certain infections. This plant generally has a more significant antibacterial effect on gram-positive bacteria. Eucalyptus was recommended for the prevention of gonorrhea in several situations, with excellent results.

Silybum marianum

One of the herbal medications used in conjunction with conventional treatment to treat STDs is Silybum marianum. The herb S. marianum is a great choice for eliminating such STDs since it contains large amounts of silymarin, a natural ingredient that may kill T. vaginalis. Additionally, this medication is often used to enhance the body's immunological response, aiding in the fight against the parasite that causes inflammation.

Soma

Soma is regarded as one of the most potent natural and herbal remedies as well as a home remedy for the treatment of STDs due to its strong antibacterial properties. The antibacterial and anti-inflammatory benefits of leaves, tree bark, roots, and soma fruit are undeniable, and they may treat illnesses like gonorrhea and syphilis. Additionally, Soma creates saponin, a plant molecule (phytochemical) that boosts the immune system, fights pathogens, and promotes bodily regeneration.

Herpes Cure

Dr. Sebi passed away from pneumonia in 2016 while incarcerated in Honduras at 82. Dr. Sebi was exposed to the elements because of the jail's poor living conditions and inadequate insulation.

The adult children of Dr. Sebi continue to support their father's health philosophy, which emphasizes the value of STD prevention via safe sex. They have given a ton of interviews since his passing to discuss who their father was, and they always emphasize the value of using condoms and maintaining a nutritious diet.

What We Need to Know About Dr. Sebi's Diet?

Due to Sebi's strict restrictions on animal-based proteins, dairy, eggs, and even soy, the diet is severely low in protein. He also restricts a lot of legumes and beans. The only foods with any protein are a few "natural rising grains," walnuts, hemp seeds, and Brazil nuts. It could be exceedingly difficult to fulfill these goods' nutritional needs on your own.

The primary building block of every cell in the body, protein aids in tissue construction and repair. The human body needs protein. Protein is a crucial component of cartilage, bones, organs, flesh, blood, and other body tissues. Limiting meal types and macronutrients may lead to poor nutrition and malnutrition. While certain fruits and vegetables are supported, it oddly restricts a lot. For example, it offers cherry or plum tomatoes but not any other varieties. Other goods he regulates include iceberg salad and shiitake mushrooms, making the diet far more restrictive and difficult to follow.

Sebi's main emphasis is on his supplements, which make grand promises that they would "revitalize and activate intercellular growth" and "quicken the healing process." Some packets cost upwards of $1,500 and include no information about the nutrients or amount. This makes it tough to understand what exactly his supplements are made of and how much you get from his unique mixtures. Sebi is not a practitioner in any way, shape, or form, and any research does not support his claims and recommendations. Its excessively strict dietary guidelines encourage the elimination of substantial food categories and macronutrients that might have significant health effects and, not to mention, could interfere negatively with other foods. To know the truth and ensure that any diet you follow is supported by research, it's critical to avoid falling into a dieting conspiracy.

The following are some potential health benefits of plant-based diets:

1. Weight loss: A 2015 study found that compared to other less restrictive diets, a vegan diet produced higher weight reduction. Participants dropped up to 7.5 percent of their body weight after six months on a vegan diet.

2. Appetite control: A 2016 study of young male participants revealed that they experience more happiness after ingesting a plant-based meal made up of peas and beans than after consuming a meat-based meal.

3. Altering the microbiome: The bacteria in the stomach are collectively referred to as the "microbiome." A 2019 study found that a plant-based diet may alter the microbiome in a way that reduces the risk of illness. However, further research would be required to verify this.

4. Lower risk of illness: According to 2017 research, a plant-based diet reduces the risk of cardiovascular disease by 39% and the likelihood of developing metabolic syndrome and diabetes mellitus by 50%.

4.1 Is it Safe?

If they follow this diet, they may benefit from seeing a doctor who could recommend additional nutrients.

The B-12 vitamin

The diet of Dr. Sebi may cause a vitamin B-12 deficit. A person may be able to prevent this by consuming vitamins and meals that have been fortified. The creation of DNA and the preservation of nerve and blood cells depends on vitamin B-12, an essential nutrient. In general, older folks and those who choose a vegan or vegetarian diet are more likely to suffer from a B-12 shortage. Doctors often advise patients who don't consume animal products to take B-12 pills. Lack of B-12 may cause depression, exhaustion, and tingling in the hands and feet. Pernicious anemia, which inhibits the body from producing red blood cells that are adequately safe, is also a possibility.

Protein

Dietary protein enhances the health of the brain, bones, lungs, hormones, and DNA. According to current guidelines, women over 19 should consume a maximum of 46 grams (g) of protein daily, while men of the same age should consume 56 g. Certain items utilized

in the Dr. Sebi diet include protein. For instance, 100.0 g of hulled hemp seeds have 32.0 g of protein, compared to 16.7 g in 100 g of walnuts. Comparatively, 16.8 g of nutrients are present in 100 g of oven-roasted chicken breast.

However, several plant protein sources, like rice, lentils, and soy, are not allowed in the Dr. Sebi diet. A person will need to eat an exceptionally high volume of legal protein sources to meet routine needs. According to research, it's important to have enough amino acids, the building blocks of protein, if you want to consume a wide range of plant foods. Adopting the Dr. Sebi diet might make this difficult.

Omega-3 fatty acids

Omega-3 fatty acids are necessary for cell membranes to function. They endorse:

- The health of the head, heart, and eye
- Power
- The immune response

The Dr. Sebi diet includes foods like hemp seeds and walnuts that are rich in plant-based omega-3s. However, the liver is more adept at extracting these acids from animal sources. According to 2019 research, a vegan diet supplies little to no omega-3 fatty acids unless the person takes a supplement. The Dr. Sebi diet will benefit someone who takes an omega-3 supplement.

4.2 Herbal Medicine

Herbal medicine is defined as "the knowledge, skills, and methods based on the philosophies, beliefs, and relationships unique to many nations, applied in the health preservation and health prevention, assessment, augmentation, or treatment of the mental and physical problem" Traditional medicine has several various structures. The environment governs each action and theory, particular circumstances, and geographic region in which it originated. Regardless of the underlying condition or sickness the patient has, the focus is often on their overall health, and using herbs is a key component of many traditional medicine regimens.

Traditional Chinese medicine has been a key example of how classical and acquired knowledge is used via a methodical approach to modern medical treatment (TCM). TCM has a more than 3,000-year history. The Devine Farmer's Classic of Herbalism, the world's oldest known herbal treatise, was written in China around 2000 years ago. However, the scientifically documented and accumulated herbal information has developed into multiple herbal pharmacopeias and countless monographs on specific plants.

Treatment and diagnosis are based on a balanced understanding of the illness and its repercussions, as symbolized by the Yin-Yang combination. In contrast to Yang, who represents the sky, masculinity, and heat, yin represents femininity, the soil, and ice. The interactions between the five elements that make up the world—wood, water, metal, earth, and fire—are influenced by yin and Yang. The 12 meridians that TCM practitioners control transport and direct energy (Qi) through a body to varying degrees of Yang and yin. TCM

is a growing practice used to promote health and ward off and prevent sickness. TCM involves various activities, although traditional treatments and organic components are key.

The development and mass production of chemically produced medications throughout the last century has changed healthcare in several parts of the world. However, in wealthy nations, sizable portions of the populace also rely on traditional doctors and herbal treatments as the main form of therapy. For their medical requirements, up to 90% of people in Africa and 70% of people in India use conventional medicine. Over 90% of state hospitals in China include traditional medicine departments, and conventional medicine makes up about 40% of all healthcare services offered. However, herbal treatments are not only practiced in developing countries. During the last 20 years, ethnobotanicals have greatly increased the public interest in herbal remedies in industrialized nations.

The most common reasons for using natural remedies are that they are more widely available, more closely align with the patient's lifestyle, allay fears about the negative effects of synthetic (artificial) drugs, satisfy the need for more individualized healthcare, and enable a more thorough community approach to health records. The major uses of herbal medicines are to improve human health, treat chronic illnesses, and prevent serious illnesses. However, as contemporary infectious illnesses and advanced malignancies are managed clinically, natural therapies are becoming increasingly popular. Natural medicines, in contrast, are widely acknowledged, non-toxic, and beneficial.

Herbal medicine is a vital component of health care, whether a person needs it or not, whether they have access to allopathic treatment physically or financially. Its global market is expanding.

Currently, herbs are used to treat various conditions, including heart disease, obesity, asthma, anxiety, and prostate diseases, as well as chronic and severe illnesses, disorders, and concerns. In China in 2003, the strategy for containing and treating SARS (severe acute respiratory syndrome) relied heavily on conventional natural therapies. The African flower is a traditional herbal remedy that has been used for a very long time in Africa to treat HIV-related illnesses. In Europe, natural remedies are still popular. It is common to find herbal extracts, teas, and essential oils at pharmacies that offer prescription pharmaceuticals in most industrialized nations, with France and Germany topping total European purchasing.

Herbs and seeds may be produced and consumed in various forms, including entire herbs, teas, syrups, lavender oil, ointments, salves, rubbers, pills, and capsules containing a powdered dry extract of a raw herb form. In addition to vinegar (extracts of acetic acid), alcoholic extracts, hot water extracts (tisanes), extended boiling extracts, often bark and roots (decoctions), and cold plant infusions, there are other types of plant and herb extracts. There isn't much detail, and the components in herbal products often vary greatly across batches and producers.

There are many different plant species, and their compounds are diverse. The majority are secondary plant metabolites that include aromatic compounds, the majority of which are phenols or phenolic compounds that have had oxygen added, such as tannins. They include a lot of antioxidants.

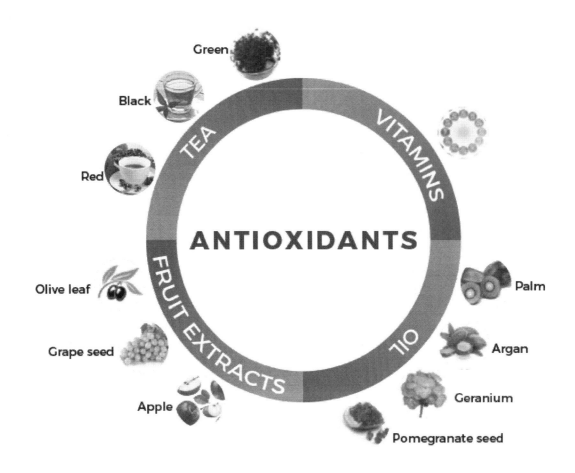

4.3 Nutritional Guide Food Recommendations:

1   Amaranth greens, mango, bell peppers, chayote, cucumber, garbanzo beans, kale, Izote, lettuce, Nopales, okra, olives, onions, sea vegetables, squash, zucchini, tomatoes (only cherry and plum), tomatillo, purslane, and wild arugula are among the veggies.

2   Fruits: papayas, oranges, strawberries, bananas, berries (all types except cranberries), elderberries, cantaloupe, lemons, mango, currants, dates, figs, grapes (seeded), melons (seeded), tamarind, peaches, plums, pears, prickly pears, prunes, and grapes (seeded) (seeded)

3   Olive oil, coconut oil, sesame oil, hemp oil, grape seed oil, and avocado oil should not be cooked.

BOOK 15:

Dr. Sebi Alkaline-Based Plant-Diet

Dr. Sebi is a well-known herbalist who has successfully treated many patients with various conditions, including aids, asthma, herpes, hair loss, fibroids, hypertension, body aches, and others. He said that acidity and mucus are what cause the ailments. As a result, regular use of natural botanical remedies will help a diseased body detoxify and effectively cleanse itself by returning it to its normal alkaline state. He asserted that only an acidic environment might cause sickness.

He thought that eating some foods and avoiding others would purify the body, keeping it in an alkaline state to reduce illness risk and impact—starting to eat an alkaline-based plant-based diet helps with cancer treatment. The formula's essential tenet is that no disease or parasite can survive outside of an acidic environment.

Dr. Sebi further noted that several unprocessed fruits and vegetables are packed with elements that may revitalize and purify the body at the intracellular and intercellular levels.

Dr. Sebi's alkaline diet incorporates a variety of guidelines, like:

- Consume just the meals listed in the handbook.
- Consume 1 gallon of pure spring water each day.
- Steer clear of alcohol, animal-derived goods, and hybrid diets.
- Quit using the microwave, which "kills your supper."

- Keep away from canned and seedless fruit.

1. Feed vegetables and raw fruits. Many of which can be found below:

Vegetables

Wild arugula, bell peppers, avocado, cucumber, dandelions, amaranth greens, Mexican squash (chayote), Inle cactus flower, onions, olives, okra, sea vegetables, tomato (only plum and cherry), tomatillo turnip greens, squash, purslane (verdelage), zucchini, and watercress are some of the other ingredients.

Fruits

Mid-size bananas or burru (original banana), Elderberries of many varieties but no cranberries, Dates with currants, seeded grapes, figs, and cherries.

2. Limit starch and sugar.

The fact is that sugar feeds some types of disease-causing cells in the body, which is essential to our everyday survival. Sugar is essential for providing food to bodily cells. Consuming glucose or converting it from carbs is necessary for cells to function.

Yes, sugar feeds cancer cells; this is a fact that stands at the heart of the sugar and cancer debate. However, it provides them the same energy as all other bodily cells. An unhealthy sugar craving might lead to several health issues, including a higher risk of developing several malignancies.

In the same way that sugar may be converted into fat when necessary, the body can also do the opposite and treat sugar as fat when it is not required.

According to Professor Aranda, those who consume more sugar are more likely to become overweight or obese, which is a risk factor for developing cancer.

2. Drink a gallon (not alkaline water) of fresh spring water.

6.4 For the Healing Process

Cleanse the body

The body should be detoxified on an intracellular level to cleanse the body's cells. Remove the mucus.

Revitalize the body

The body would then begin to regenerate, leading to rejuvenation. (Eat a lot of sea moss and iron).

Begin with a detox

According to the research, regeneration occurs in the stomach, implying that alkaline diets and colon cleansing are necessary. To cleanse the colon, use herbs. Another way to clear it up is to go without food for at least three to thirty days. The effect will be more pronounced the longer the fast. However, we shall briefly discuss the benefits of fasting in the coming chapters. Juice, water, or smoothies should be consumed.

To get rid of cancer says Dr. Sebi, the intestines, kidneys, gall bladder, lymph nodes, liver, and eyes must be cleaned.

6.5 Foods and Herbs

Later, Sebi focused on African plants and herbs and hypothesized that an excess of plants, especially naturally alkaline fruits and vegetables, might purge the body and cause it to become alkaline.

These alkaline plants carry out their functions by eliminating harmful substances stored throughout the body and allowing the rejuvenation of key minerals depleted by the body's acid content.

Some amazing alkaline foods have surprising characteristics that kill cancer cells. There are several groups:

Cleansing herbs

1. Burdock root: This may be used to cleanse the liver and lymphatic system.

Dandelion: The kidney and gall bladder are cleaned.

3. Mullein: Promotes lymphatic flow in the neck and chest and detoxifies the lungs.

4. Chaparral: Removes heavy metals from the blood and gall bladder while clearing the lymphatic system.

5. Elderberry: Removes mucus from the upper respiratory tract and lungs.

Eucalyptus: Use steam to cleanse the skin.

7. Cascara Sagrada: Triggers muscle spasms that aid in moving excrement through the colon.

8. Rhubarb root is an effective laxative that supports the digestive system.

Revitalizing herbs

1. Sarsaparilla root: The source of the most iron. Being able to oxygenate your blood and cells will aid in your recovery while you work to recover from your sickness. (Jamaican is suggested.)

2. Sea moss (Irish moss): This plant contains 92 to 102 minerals that the body needs. (Wildcrafted is preferred)

3. Pao Pereira: Cancer cells have been scientifically shown to be lethal in the brain, pancreatic, breast, kidney, and other organs. Possess the capacity to reduce tumors, in contrast to the toxicity of radiation and chemotherapy that you would undergo. Even if you do not currently have cancer, this herb is preventative. Herbal alkaloids toxicly damage some cancer cells, yet healthy body cells are unaffected. It easily crosses the blood-brain barrier and attaches itself to brain cancer cells. Additionally, it purifies the blood and liver. Along with chemotherapy and radiation treatment, it is thought to be used in treating many forms of cancer and is often designed to boost the immune system.

4. Soursop: 10,000 times more effective than chemotherapy in killing cancer cells. It lessens the size of the tumor, eradicates cancerous cells, and boosts the immune system's defenses.

5. CBD Oil: A Proven Cancer Treatment

6. Anamu (Guinea Hen Weed) is ideal for destroying cells.

6.6 Anticancer Properties of Nigella sativa

Nigella sativa, sometimes known as black cumin, has a long history of usage in medicine. It was used in ancient Egypt, Greece, Africa, and the Middle East. It originated in South East Asia. Islam regards it as one of the finest methods for healing medicine. It is a blooming plant whose taste comes from the seeds. It has undergone extensive in vivo and in vitro investigation. Proapoptotic, antiproliferative, cytotoxic, antioxidant, anti-I-metastatic, anti-mutagenic, and N.K. properties are present in black cumin. Its impact on different cancer cell lines and primary cancer cells is strengthened by its cytotoxic activity.

- N. sativa's active ingredients are beneficial for treating various diseases, including cancer.

- Natural oils, proteins, saponin, and alkaloids are present in the seed. The N Sativa oil contains four substances that are fundamental to pharmacology: dithymoquinone (DTQ), Thymol (THY), thymohydroquinone (THQ), Thymoquinone, and (T.Q.)

Blood cancer

T.Q. has antiproliferative activity in HL-60 cells and 518A2 melanoma, derivatives of T.Q., in human myeloblastic leukemia HL-60 cells. We looked examined 6-alkyl residues carrying terpene ends. Apoptosis was shown to be caused by the products and was linked to DNA laddering, a loss in mitochondrial membrane function, and a little increase in oxygen reactive species. Murine leukemia P388 cells increased apoptosis after receiving a dosage of -hederin.

Breast cancer

Both alcoholic and aqueous extracts of N. sativa successfully inactivated breast cancer MCF-7 cells in a test tube.

Colon cancer

T.Q. is antineoplastic and proapoptotic against colon cancer cells from the HCT116 line.

Cancer of the pancreas

In pancreatic ductal adenocarcinoma cells, T.Q., an important component of N. sativa oil extract, mediates apoptosis and inhibits proliferation (PDA). They also presented T.Q. as a new pro-inflammatory pathway inhibitor, offering a convincing strategy that combines proapoptotic and anti-inflammatory modes of action.

Hepatic cancer

By effectively enhancing the growth of glutathione transferase and quinone reductase, oral T.Q. administration makes the substance a potent preventative against chemical carcinogenesis and hepatic cancer toxicity.

Lung cancer

N. Sativa has a protective function against methyl nitrosourea (MNU)-induced oxidative damage, inflammatory response, and carcinogenesis in the lungs, skin, and colon.

Although N. sativa's anticancer properties have been known for thousands of years, this important herbal remedy has just recently undergone a rigorous clinical evaluation. Further research should be emphasized since it is a stable endeavor. Several researchers think that traditional medical care might be included in novel cancer therapies, and N. Sativa's research may be used to investigate novel anticancer strategies and methodologies.

BOOK16: Dr. Sebi:

Sacred Medicinal Plants

Several plants hold sacred significance in Native American herbalism. These plants are revered not only for their healing properties but also for their spiritual and ceremonial uses. Examples of such sacred medicinal plants include sage, cedar, sweetgrass, tobacco, and many others. These plants are often used in purification rituals, prayer ceremonies, and for fostering a connection with the spiritual world.

6.4 The Alchemy of Healing

Native American herbalism goes beyond the physical aspects of healing and embraces the concept of alchemy, where healing is viewed as a transformational process. It involves not only the treatment of symptoms but also a deep exploration of the root causes of illness, which may include emotional and spiritual imbalances. The alchemical approach seeks to restore harmony and alignment with nature and the universe.

6.5 Herbal Rituals and Ceremonies

Herbal rituals and ceremonies are integral to Native American healing practices. These ceremonies often involve the use of medicinal plants, drumming, singing, and dancing to create a sacred and healing space. Rituals may vary among tribes and communities, but they all share the common intention of promoting healing, unity, and connection with the spiritual realm.

6.6 Respecting Traditional Knowledge

As we explore the wisdom of Native American herbalism and alchemy, it is essential to approach this knowledge with deep respect and reverence. Traditional knowledge is a precious legacy that must be preserved and honored. When incorporating Native American healing practices into our lives, it is crucial to do so with humility, cultural sensitivity, and a willingness to learn from the wisdom of the indigenous peoples.

Native American herbalism and alchemy offer profound insights into the interconnectedness of all life and the power of plants to heal and transform. By embracing the wisdom of these ancient traditions, we can cultivate a deeper connection with nature and our own inner healing potential. As we continue on our journey of herbal medicine, let us honor and carry forward the sacred knowledge of Native American healers, integrating their wisdom into our modern approach to holistic healing.

Essential Oils - Nature's Aromatic Healers

Essential oils have been treasured for their therapeutic properties and captivating fragrances for thousands of years. Derived from aromatic plants, these precious oils carry the essence of nature's healing power. In this chapter, we will delve into the fascinating world of essential oils, exploring their extraction methods, therapeutic uses, and safety considerations. As we unlock the secrets of these aromatic healers, we will discover their potential to support physical, emotional, and spiritual well-being.

7.1 Understanding Essential Oils

Essential oils are highly concentrated plant extracts obtained through various methods, such as steam distillation, cold pressing, or solvent extraction. These potent oils capture the plant's aromatic compounds, which contain the essence and medicinal properties of the plant. Each essential oil boasts a unique chemical composition, giving it distinct therapeutic benefits.

7.2 The Science of Aromatherapy

Aromatherapy is the art and science of using essential oils to enhance overall well-being. When inhaled or applied to the skin, essential oils interact with the body's limbic system, influencing emotions, memory, and mood. Aromatherapy is a complementary healing modality that can be used alongside conventional medicine to promote relaxation, reduce stress, and support emotional balance.

7.3 Popular Essential Oils and Their Uses

There is a vast array of essential oils, each with its own therapeutic properties and applications. We will explore some of the most popular essential oils and their uses:

Lavender (Lavandula angustifolia): Renowned for its calming and soothing properties, lavender is commonly used to promote relaxation, improve sleep quality, and alleviate anxiety.

Peppermint (Mentha piperita): Peppermint essential oil is known for its invigorating and refreshing effects. It can help ease headaches, relieve digestive discomfort, and boost energy levels.

Tea Tree (Melaleuca alternifolia): With powerful antiseptic and antimicrobial properties, tea tree oil is a staple in natural skin care remedies. It is beneficial for treating acne, fungal infections, and insect bites.

Eucalyptus (Eucalyptus globulus): This oil is revered for its respiratory benefits. Eucalyptus can alleviate congestion, soothe coughs, and support respiratory health.

Chamomile (Matricaria chamomilla): Chamomile essential oil is prized for its calming effects. It can help ease tension, promote relaxation, and aid in managing stress and insomnia.

Frankincense (Boswellia carterii): A sacred oil in many cultures, frankincense is renowned for its spiritual and meditative properties. It can promote a sense of grounding and connection during meditation and prayer.

7.4 Application Methods and Safety Precautions

When using essential oils, it is essential to apply them safely and appropriately. Different oils require varying dilution ratios, and some may need to be avoided during pregnancy or certain medical conditions. Common application methods include inhalation, topical application, and diffusion. We will provide detailed guidelines on how to use essential oils safely to maximize their benefits and minimize the risk of adverse reactions.

7.5 Blending Essential Oils

Creating custom blends of essential oils allows you to tailor their therapeutic effects to your specific needs and preferences. We will explore the art of blending essential oils, discussing the principles of complementary scents and the science behind creating harmonious blends. Whether you are seeking relaxation, energy, or emotional support, blending essential oils can be a creative and effective way to harness their healing potential.

7.6 Incorporating Aromatherapy into Daily Life

Aromatherapy is a versatile practice that can be easily integrated into daily life. From using essential oils in diffusers to crafting personalized body oils, bath salts, and sprays, we will provide practical tips and recipes to help you incorporate aromatherapy into your self-care routine. Discover how to create a calming bedtime ritual, an energizing morning routine, or a soothing space for meditation.

7.7 The Power of Scent and Memory

Scent has a profound impact on our memories and emotions. We will explore the connection between scent and memory, understanding how certain aromas can evoke past experiences and emotions. By harnessing the power of scent, we can use essential oils to create positive associations and support emotional healing.

Essential oils offer a treasure trove of therapeutic benefits and aromatic delights. From promoting physical healing to supporting emotional well-being, these gifts of nature have the power to enhance our lives on multiple levels. By understanding their unique properties and practicing aromatherapy with care and respect, we can harness the full potential of essential oils and embrace nature's aromatic healers as powerful allies on our journey to holistic wellness.

Herbal Remedies for Common Ailments - Nature's Healing Panacea

In this chapter, we will explore the world of herbal remedies and their time-honored tradition of healing. Herbal medicine has been practiced for centuries, drawing on the wisdom of ancient civilizations and indigenous cultures. From alleviating minor ailments to supporting overall wellness, herbs have been regarded as nature's healing panacea. Join us as we delve into the diverse world of herbal remedies, uncovering their therapeutic uses, preparation methods, and evidence-based benefits.

8.1 Understanding Herbal Medicine

Herbal medicine, also known as herbalism, is the use of plants and plant extracts to promote health and treat various ailments. It is a holistic approach that considers not only the physical symptoms but also the underlying imbalances in the body. Herbal remedies work synergistically with the body's natural healing processes, offering gentle yet potent support.

8.2 The Healing Power of Common Herbs

We will explore a selection of commonly used herbs and their therapeutic properties:

Calendula (Calendula officinalis): Known for its soothing and anti-inflammatory properties, calendula is beneficial for skin irritations, minor cuts, and burns.

Echinacea (Echinacea purpurea): A popular immune-boosting herb, echinacea can help prevent and reduce the severity of colds and flu.

Ginger (Zingiber officinale): With its warming and anti-nausea properties, ginger is an effective remedy for digestive discomfort and motion sickness.

Chamomile (Matricaria chamomilla): Chamomile's gentle calming effects make it a go-to herb for promoting relaxation and relieving stress.

Peppermint (Mentha piperita): Peppermint aids in digestion, eases headaches, and offers a refreshing and cooling sensation.

Valerian (Valeriana officinalis): A natural sedative, valerian can improve sleep quality and reduce insomnia and anxiety.

8.3 Preparing Herbal Remedies

Discover the various methods of preparing herbal remedies, such as teas, infusions, decoctions, tinctures, and herbal oils. Each preparation method extracts different constituents from the plant, making them suitable for different therapeutic purposes. We will provide step-by-step instructions for preparing herbal remedies at home, empowering you to become your own herbalist.

8.4 Evidence-Based Benefits of Herbal Medicine

While herbal remedies have a long history of traditional use, modern scientific research has also shed light on their therapeutic benefits. We will delve into the evidence-based benefits of specific herbs and explore how they can complement conventional medicine. From supporting cardiovascular health to managing stress and anxiety, we will highlight the growing body of research supporting the efficacy of herbal medicine.

8.5 Integrating Herbal Medicine with Conventional Care

Herbal medicine can be a valuable addition to conventional medical treatments. We will discuss how to integrate herbal remedies safely and effectively with conventional care, ensuring they enhance each other's benefits while avoiding potential interactions. Consultation with healthcare professionals is essential, especially when addressing chronic or severe health conditions.

8.6 Herbal Remedies for the Whole Family

Herbal medicine is suitable for individuals of all ages, from infants to the elderly. We will explore age-appropriate herbal remedies for common ailments, ensuring that the whole family can benefit from nature's healing gifts. Safety considerations and proper dosages for children and seniors will be discussed to ensure their well-being.

8.7 Growing and Cultivating Medicinal Herbs

For those with green thumbs and a passion for gardening, we will provide guidance on growing and cultivating medicinal herbs at home. Cultivating your healing garden allows you to have a readily available supply of fresh herbs for your herbal remedies, fostering a deeper connection with nature and the healing process.

Herbal remedies have stood the test of time, offering a holistic and gentle approach to healing. As we continue to explore the therapeutic properties of common herbs and their evidence-based benefits, we are reminded of the wisdom and generosity of natureEmbracing herbal medicine empowers us to take charge of our health and well-being, tapping into the abundance of nature's healing panacea. Whether you seek to alleviate common ailments or support overall wellness, herbal remedies are a timeless ally on your journey to optimal health and vitality.

Ù

Book 17:

Dr. Sebi medicinal herbs

Recipes

Sage (Salvia officinalis)

Medicinal Properties: Sage has antibacterial and anti-inflammatory properties and is used to treat sore throats, coughs, and respiratory infections.

Recipe: Sage Gargle for Sore Throat: Prepare a decoction with sage leaves in boiling water and use it for gargling once cooled. Repeat several times a day.

Lavender (Lavandula angustifolia)

Medicinal Properties: Lavender has calming and relaxing properties and is used to alleviate stress, anxiety, and insomnia.

Recipe: Lavender Essential Oil for Skin Care: Mix a few drops of lavender essential oil with a carrier oil and apply it to the skin to soothe irritations and inflammations. Also ideal for a relaxing bath.

Echinacea (Echinacea purpurea)

Medicinal Properties: Echinacea is known for boosting the immune system and is used for preventing and treating colds and infections.

Recipe: Echinacea Tincture for Immune Support: Macerate echinacea roots in alcohol for several weeks and use it as a supplement to support the immune system.

Ginseng (Panax ginseng)

Medicinal Properties: Ginseng is a natural tonic that helps improve energy, concentration, and stress resistance.

Recipe: Ginseng Tea for Energy: Pour hot water over a few slices of ginseng root and steep for 10-15 minutes. Drink in the morning for a stimulating effect.

Calendula (Calendula officinalis)

Medicinal Properties: Calendula has anti-inflammatory and soothing properties and is used to treat skin irritations and wounds.

Recipe: Calendula Salve for Skin: Prepare a calendula oil by macerating the flowers in olive oil for several weeks. Use the oil to make a salve to apply to affected areas.

Peppermint (Mentha x piperita)

Medicinal Properties: Peppermint has digestive properties and can help reduce bloating and stomach discomfort.

Recipe: Peppermint Tea for Digestion: Pour boiling water over a few peppermint leaves and steep for 5 minutes. Drink after meals to aid digestion.

Turmeric (Curcuma longa)

Medicinal Properties: Turmeric has anti-inflammatory and antioxidant properties and is used to alleviate joint pain and inflammation.

Recipe: Golden Milk with Turmeric: Mix warm almond milk with turmeric powder, black pepper, and honey. Drink to promote joint health.

Aloe Vera (Aloe barbadensis miller)

Medicinal Properties: Aloe vera has soothing properties and is used to treat burns and skin irritations.

Recipe: DIY Aloe Vera Gel: Cut an aloe vera leaf and extract the transparent gel. Apply directly to the skin to soothe irritations.

Lemon Balm (Melissa officinalis)

Medicinal Properties: Lemon balm has calming properties and can help reduce anxiety and improve mood.

Recipe: Lemon Balm Tea for Mental Well-being: Pour hot water over a few lemon balm leaves and steep for 5-7 minutes. Drink during moments of stress or agitation.

Guide to Medicinal Plants and Herbs (Continued)

St. John's Wort (Hypericum perforatum)

Medicinal Properties: St. John's Wort is used as a natural antidepressant and mood enhancer.

Recipe: St. John's Wort Infused Oil: Infuse St. John's Wort flowers in olive oil for several weeks. Use the oil topically to alleviate mild depression and nerve pain.

Valerian (Valeriana officinalis)

Medicinal Properties: Valerian is known for its sedative properties and is used to promote sleep and alleviate anxiety.

Recipe: Valerian Root Sleep Aid: Prepare a decoction with valerian root in water and drink before bedtime for a restful sleep.

Dandelion (Taraxacum officinale)

Medicinal Properties: Dandelion has diuretic properties and is used to support liver and kidney health.

Recipe: Dandelion Detox Tea: Steep dandelion leaves and roots in hot water for 10 minutes. Drink to help cleanse the body.

Elderberry (Sambucus nigra)

Medicinal Properties: Elderberry is known for its immune-boosting properties and is used to prevent and treat colds and flu.

Recipe: Elderberry Syrup for Immune Support: Boil elderberries in water, strain, and add honey. Take as a daily supplement during cold and flu season.

Garlic (Allium sativum)

Medicinal Properties: Garlic has antimicrobial properties and is used to boost the immune system and support heart health.

Recipe: Garlic Honey for Immunity: Crush garlic cloves and mix them with honey. Consume a teaspoon daily to enhance immunity.

Rosemary (Rosmarinus officinalis)

Medicinal Properties: Rosemary has antioxidant and anti-inflammatory properties and is used to improve cognitive function and digestion.

Recipe: Rosemary Oil for Hair and Scalp: Infuse rosemary leaves in olive oil for several weeks. Use the oil as a hair and scalp treatment.

Yarrow (Achillea millefolium)

Medicinal Properties: Yarrow has astringent and anti-inflammatory properties and is used to treat wounds and minor bleeding.

Recipe: Yarrow Salve for Wound Healing: Prepare a salve using yarrow-infused oil and beeswax. Apply to wounds for healing.

Nettle (Urtica dioica)

Medicinal Properties: Nettle is a natural anti-allergen and is used to alleviate seasonal allergies and hay fever.

Recipe: Nettle Leaf Tea for Allergies: Steep nettle leaves in hot water for 5 minutes. Drink to relieve allergy symptoms.

Licorice (Glycyrrhiza glabra)

Medicinal Properties: Licorice has anti-inflammatory properties and is used to soothe sore throats and digestive issues.

Recipe: Licorice Root Tea for Digestive Health: Boil licorice root in water and steep for 10 minutes. Drink to relieve digestive discomfort.

Ginger (Zingiber officinale)

Medicinal Properties: Ginger has anti-nausea and anti-inflammatory properties and is used to alleviate nausea and muscle pain.
Recipe: Ginger Infused Water for Nausea: Infuse ginger slices in water and drink to ease nausea and indigestion.

Creating Herbal Formulations

In this chapter, we will delve into the art of creating herbal formulations by combining various medicinal plants and herbs to enhance their healing properties. Formulations can be in the form of teas, tinctures, salves, oils, and more, each serving specific health purposes. Understanding the synergy between different herbs will allow you to create potent and effective remedies for various ailments.

Herbal Tea Blends

Exploring the art of herbal tea blending and how to combine different herbs to address specific health concerns.

Recipes for Relaxing Herbal Tea, Immune-Boosting Tea, Digestive Aid Tea, and more.

Herbal Tinctures and Extracts

Understanding the process of making herbal tinctures and extracts using alcohol or glycerin as solvents.

Recipes for Calming Tincture, Energy-Boosting Tincture, and Immune Support Extract.

Herbal Salves and Balms

Discovering the process of creating healing salves and balms using infused oils and beeswax.

Recipes for Healing Salve for Cuts and Scrapes, Muscle Relief Balm, and Skin Soothing Salve.

Herbal Oils and Infused Vinegars

Exploring the benefits of herbal oils and vinegars and how to create them for culinary and medicinal use.

Recipes for Herbal-Infused Olive Oil, Rosemary-Infused Vinegar, and Lavender-Infused Sunflower Oil.

Herbal Capsules and Pills

Learning how to encapsulate powdered herbs for convenient and controlled dosing.

Recipes for Herbal Sleep Aid Capsules, Immune Support Pills, and Digestive Health Capsules.

BOOK 18:

Dr. Sebi's: Anti-Inflammatory

An anti-inflammatory diet is one of the most talked-about diets right now for a reason, but first, you need to learn what inflammation is. Many people associate inflammation with swollen or reddened skin after stubbing their toes. Inflammation can be seen in these two ways, but there's more going on.

As a component of the body's immunological reaction, inflammation develops. Inflammatory cells are sent to the rescue if your body is battling an illness or damage. Swelling, redness, or occasional discomfort are all symptoms of this condition. Natural and acceptable behavior.

That is, as far as your body remains under control. When inflammation persists and does not go away, the narrative shifts. Several health problems are associated with chronic inflammation, such as heart disease, Alzheimer's, type 2 diabetes, and cancer.

Fortunately, you have some influence over the inflammation levels. You may be more susceptible to inflammation if you smoke, are obese or overweight, or drink to excess, such as excessively. According to some specialists, it's possible to lessen inflammation levels by altering your diet rather than using the medicine. It's also a good idea to only use medicine for chronic pain if it's required since many medications have unpleasant side effects, such as tiredness, fogginess, and memory loss.

An official anti-inflammatory diet does not exist that specifies precisely what, how often, and when one should consume. On the other hand, anti-inflammatory food is about consuming foods that have been proven to reduce inflammation and exclude those found to increase it.

Anti-inflammatory diet advocate Brittany Scanniello, RD, recommends thinking of the meal as a way of life instead of a diet. An anti-inflammatory meal, according to her, "helps to lessen or limit your bodies' low-grade inflammation."

Fruits and vegetables are an essential part of any healthy diet, as are complex carbs like whole-grain pieces of bread and pasta and a limited amount of dairy.

Are you keen to know more about anti-inflammatory diets and how they might help you avoid certain diseases? Onwards!

Anti-inflammatory diet What to know

As a symptom of sickness, inflammation may serve as a shield to keep the body safe from further damage. It's a vital aspect of the recovery process in most situations.

On the other hand, some individuals suffer from a medical problem that impairs the immune system's function. Persistent or recurring low-level inflammation may be the result of this dysfunction.

Rheumatoid arthritis, Psoriasis, and asthma are just a few disorders that may cause chronic inflammation. There's evidence to suggest that changing one's diet might assist with the symptoms.

An anti-inflammatory meal includes fruits and veggies, lean protein, whole grains, omega-3 fatty acids, healthy fats, and spices. Processed foods and alcohol are discouraged or limited in this diet.

An anti-inflammatory meal is more of a way of eating than a program. Anti-inflammatory meals include such like the Mediterranean & DASH diets.

1.1 What is an anti-inflammatory diet?

A diet low in processed foods is recommended for those with inflammatory diseases.

Certain substances in meals have the potential to either cause or aggravate inflammation. Meals high in sugar and processed ingredients may have this impact, although whole, healthy foods are far less likely to do so.

Fresh vegetables and fruits are key components of an anti-inflammatory meal. Antioxidants are abundant in plant-based meals. On the other hand, some meals may set off the production of radicals in the body. Foods fried in repeatedly heated oil are one example of this.

The chemicals in food known as dietary antioxidants assist the body in eliminating free radicals. When somebody functions, such as metabolism, produce free radicals, they end up in the environment. However, the number of free radicals within the body may be increased by external causes like stress or tobacco usage.

Cell damage is possible when free radicals are present. A variety of disorders may be aggravated or caused by this kind of damage.

Antioxidants that assist the body to eliminate this harmful comb are produced naturally, although dietary antioxidants are also beneficial.

Foods high in antioxidants are preferred over those that raise free radicals during an anti-inflammatory lifestyle.

1.2 Types of an anti-inflammatory diet

Anti-inflammatory concepts are already prevalent in many ketogenic diets.

Both the Mediterranean & the DASH diets, for instance, contain heart-healthy fats, fresh fruits, vegetables, seafood, and whole grains.

A Mediterranean diet, including its emphasis on plant-based meals including heart-healthy oils, may be able to minimize the impacts of inflammation upon your cardiovascular system.

1.3 Who can help?

Chronic inflammation exacerbates many diseases, which may be countered by following an anti-inflammatory lifestyle.

Inflammation is present in one of the following conditions:

- Psoriasis
- Asthma
- Rheumatoid arthritis
- Eosinophilic esophagitis

- Colitis

- Crohn's disease

- Inflammatory bowel diseases

- Hashimoto's thyroiditis

- Lupus

- Metabolic syndrome

Several disorders are known as metabolic syndrome, comprising type-2 diabetes, hypertension, obesity, & heart disease.

Inflammation, according to researchers, is a factor in each of these conditions. People with metabolic syndrome might benefit from an anti-inflammatory lifestyle.

Antioxidant-rich diets could also help lower the chance of developing some types of cancer.

1.4 Foods to eat

To combat inflammation, eat a diet rich in anti-inflammatory foods.

- Are abundant in nutrient

- Contain nourishing fats

- Provide a variety of antioxidants

Inflammation-fighting foods include:

- Fruits, including strawberries, blueberries, cherries, and blackberries

- Vegetables, including broccoli, kale, and spinach

- Fiber

- Beans

- Seeds and nuts

- Olive oil and olives

- moderately or raw, cooked veggies

- legumes, including lentils

- spices, including turmeric and ginger

- herbs

- prebiotics and probiotics

- tea

It's crucial to keep in mind:

There isn't a single meal that can improve someone's health. It's important to consume a wide range of nutritious foods.

The greatest ingredients are those made with just fresh, basic components. Foods might lose some of their nutritional value during processing.

Consumers should scrutinize premade food labeling. However, although cocoa is a wonderful option, cocoa frequently also contains fat and sugar. Cocoa

Antioxidants & other nutrients may be found in plenty on a colorful plate. Vegetables and fruit of various hues should be included in your diet.

1.5 Foods to avoid

People on anti-inflammatory dietary should steer clear of or consume as little of the following as possible:

- processed foods

- foods including added salt or sugar

- unhealthful oils

- processed carbs that are present in white pasta, white bread, & a variety of baked goods

- processed snack meals, including crackers chips

- premade desserts, including ice cream cookies, and candy

- excess alcohol

In addition, people might find it advantageous to limit their intake of the following:

Gluten: When gluten is consumed, it causes an inflammatory response in certain individuals. A gluten-free diet has pros and cons, but it's not for everyone. A person's symptoms might be alleviated by avoiding gluten for some time to determine whether it helps.

Nightshades: Some persons with inflammatory disorders have flare-ups while eating nightshade plants like eggplants, peppers, tomatoes, and potatoes. Little data supports this claim; however, people may check whether their symptoms improve by eliminating nightshades from their diet for two to three weeks.

Carbohydrates: Even when the carbohydrates are good for you, several pieces of evidence suggest that a high-carb diet might increase inflammation in certain individuals. Sweet potatoes & whole grains, for example, are good antioxidant and nutritional providers despite their carbohydrate content.

1.6 Can a vegetarian diet reduce inflammation?

People who want to minimize inflammation may find it helpful to follow a vegetarian diet. The review's authors evaluated data from 40 papers in 2019. In the end, they found that vegetarians had lower levels of inflammatory markers.

There were 268 participants in research conducted in 2017 that looked at the dietary data of either Lacto-ovo vegetarians or nonvegetarians. According to the study's results, eating animal products may raise the risk of chronic inflammation & insulin resistance.

Lower levels of inflammation may be a fundamental advantage of a vegan diet, according to a previous study from 2014.

1.7 Anti-inflammatory diet tips

It might be difficult to make the switch to a new diet, but these suggestions can help:

- Select healthy snacks & a wide range of fruits and veggies when you go grocery shopping.
- Substitute fast food dinners with cooked lunches as you become used to them.
- Mineral water may be used instead of soda & other caloric sweeteners.

- Inquiring about nutritional supplements including multivitamin or cod liver oil with your doctor

- Including 30 mins of medium physical activity each day in your schedule.

- It's important to have appropriate sleep hygiene since a lack of sleep may exacerbate inflammatory conditions.

1.8 Takeaway

Rheumatoid arthritis, for example, may benefit from an anti-inflammatory food, which reduces inflammation & alleviates symptoms.

The anti-inflammatory meal is no single; however, a diet rich in fresh fruits, whole grains, vegetables, and healthy fats may help control inflammation.

Anyone with an inflammatory chronic medical condition should speak with their doctor about the optimal food for them.

1.9. 11 Ways to Make the Most of An Anti-Inflammatory Diet + A Food List

Lowering inflammation may be advantageous if you're trying to eat healthy for the long run. Debilitating chronic diseases, including rheumatoid arthritis, osteoarthritis, heart and brain disease, & dementia and Alzheimer's and Parkinson's, are all exacerbated or made worse by chronic inflammation in the body.

Anti-inflammatory diets may help guard against some illnesses, but they may also help slow down the aging process by regulating blood sugar & improving metabolism. Here are a few of the favorite dietary hacks, as well as some of the favorite anti-inflammatory meals.

1.10 Anti-inflammatory diet tips.

For the best results with an anti-inflammatory meal, follow these guidelines:

Fiber intake should be increased to almost 25 g a day.

The natural anti-inflammatory phytonutrients present in vegetables, fruits, and whole foods may help decrease inflammation when consumed with a high fiber diet.

Fruits, Whole grains, and vegetables are good sources of fiber. Whole grains like barley and oats, vegetables including okra & eggplant, fruits including bananas (3 g of fiber per banana), & blueberries are excellent sources of fiber (3.5 g of fiber per cup).

Aim for a daily fruit & vegetable intake of at least nine servings.

Half a cup of cooked fruits or vegetables, or a cup of raw leafy vegetables, is considered one "serving."

Increase the health benefits of cooked fruits & vegetables by adding anti-inflammatory spices and herbs like turmeric and ginger.

Every week, consume four servings of alliums & crucifers.

There are many different types of alliums & crucifers, but some of the most common include onions and garlic. Other cruciferous vegetables include broccoli & cauliflower.

Consuming an average of 4 servings every week may reduce your cancer risk thanks to their high levels of antioxidants. Consuming a garlic clove a day is suggested if you enjoy the flavor.

10.0% of your caloric intake should be from saturated fat.

Reduce your risk of cardiovascular disease by eating fewer calories with saturated fat (approximately 20 g per 2,000 calf).

Marinated with spices, herbs, and acidic raw fruit drinks to minimize the formation of harmful chemicals during cooking.

Eat a lot of omega-3-rich meals.

Anecdotal evidence shows that omega-3 fatty acid has anti-inflammatory properties, and it may help decrease the chance of developing chronic illnesses, including cancer, heart disease, and arthritis.

Eat many omega-3-rich foods like walnuts, flax meal, & various beans, such as kidney, navy, and soy, to get the most benefit. In addition, it is advised to take an omega-3 supplement of high quality.

Use fat-rich oils in place of low-fat ones.

Fat is necessary for the body, but only eat fat if it has health advantages for you.

Anti-inflammatory properties may be found in olive oils (organic is preferred). Expeller-pressed sunflower, High-oleic, & safflower oil are further alternatives.

Eat healthful snacks two times a day, preferably in the middle of the day.

As a rule, fruit, unsweetened or plain Greek-style yogurt, carrots, celery sticks, or nuts including almonds, pistachios, and walnut are good options for a healthy snack.

Stay away from highly processed meals and sweets.

Inflammation occurs throughout your body when foods rich in fructose syrup or salt are consumed.

Refined sugars & artificial sweeteners should be avoided at all costs. According to research, increased insulin tolerance, elevated uric acid & hypertension levels, and an increased fatty liver risk disease are all risks associated with eating too much fructose.

Reduce or eliminate trans fats from your diet.

Studies show that persons who consume foods rich in trans-fat possess elevated amounts of protein C-reactive, a bioindicator for inflammation. This is why the FDA mandated in 2006 required food producers to indicate trans fats in nutrition labels.

Carefully read labels & avoid items with the terms "hydrogenated" or "partial hydrogenated oils" as a rule of the thumb. Shortenings, crackers, margarine, and cookies include trans fats in varying amounts.

Spices & phytonutrient-rich fruit may be used to sweeten & flavor meals.

Phytonutrients abound in most fruits & veggies. Try adding apricots, berries, apples, & even carrots to your meals to sweeten them naturally.

You may also use anti-inflammatory spices to flavor savory dishes. Some examples of these include cloves, cinnamon, thyme, turmeric, rosemary, and other anti-inflammatory herbs and spices.

BOOK 19:

COOKBOOK

Best anti-inflammatory food list.

There was a plethora of info on anti-inflammatory diets just now. Here's a full list to go over the upcoming time you go to the supermarket, though, to grab all your go-to items in a single place:

Vegetables

- onions
- Okra
- Scallions
- Garlic
- Carrots
- Broccoli
- Cabbage
- Leek
- Cauliflower
- Brussels sprouts
- Mustard greens
- Celery

Fruits

- Blueberries
- Apples
- Bananas
- Berries
- Apricots

Whole grains

- Oatmeal
- Barley

Nuts, seeds, & legumes

- Walnuts
- Flax
- Kidney beans
- Navy beans
- Almonds
- Soybeans

- Pistachios

Herbs & spices

- Ginger
- Cloves
- Turmeric

- Cinnamon
- Thyme
- Rosemary
- Sage

1.12 Foods to avoid on an anti-inflammatory diet.

Along with eating enough anti-inflammatory meals, you should also cut out substances that might be causing inflammation in the body. The following is a list of items that are strongly advised against eating:

- Corn syrup High fructose
- Foods with High sodium
- Artificial sweeteners
- Refined sugar
- Partially Hydrogenated or hydrogenated oils

The 1st step toward a healthier, stronger body is to include more good anti-inflammatory meals and reduce unhealthy ones.

Breakfast Recipes

1. Kale Pineapple Smoothie

Prep Time: 3 mins, Cook Time: 1 min, Serving: 2

Ingredients

- 2 cups kale leaves chopped stems removed lightly packed
- ¾ cup vanilla almond unsweetened milk
- 1 frozen banana medium sliced into chunks
- ¼ cup of plain Greek yogurt non-fat
- ¼ cup of pineapple pieces frozen
- 2 tbsp peanut butter crunchy or creamy
- 1 to 3 tsp honey for taste

Instructions

1. As in order given, combine the following ingredients: kale; banana; almond milk; yogurt; peanut butter pineapple; and honey.

2. Make sure to blend everything well until it's smooth. Increase the amount of milk as necessary to get the required consistency. Please take pleasure in it at your earliest convenience.

Nutritional Facts: Cal: 228, Carb 29 g, Fat: 10 g, Protein: 11g

2. Quinoa Porridge with Chai-Infused Vanilla

Prep time: 5 mins, Cook time: 10 min, Servings: 2

Ingredients

- Dry quinoa 1 cup (pref organic)

- Water 2 cups (pref alkaline)

- Cinnamon 1 stick (or 1/2 tsp)

- Ground ginger 1 1/2 tsp/ finely grated fresh root ginger 1 "piece

- Ground nutmeg 1/2 tsp (pref fresh grated)

- Coconut cream/milk 1/2 cup

- lemon skin grated 1/2 (or lime)

- Vanilla bean pod/vanilla essence 1

- Assorted nuts Sprinkle and seeds

- Coconut yogurt optional

- Cloves ground optional

- Grated apple 1 optional

Instructions

- Cook the quinoa according to the package instructions.

- If the quinoa has been cooked and drained, return it to the pan and whisk in the chai spices (ginger, cinnamon, nutmeg, and cloves if using a mortar and pestle), then add the coconut cream/milk and scrape in the vanilla pod (add the vanilla essence, drop or 2)

- Depending on how thick and creamy you want, you may use either cream or milk.

- When it's ready, shred in the apple right at the end while you're using it.

- Transfer to a dish and serve warm. To serve, grate the lemon peel over the top and sprinkle with cinnamon (extra ground). Lastly, add the nuts and seeds (sesame seeds are recommended).

- As an indulgent option, a spoonful of coconut yogurt should be served. It has an alkaline pH.

Nutrition Facts Per Serving: Calories 516 | fat 19 g, Carb 55 g, protein 12 g

3. Supercharged Scrambled Eggplant

Prep Time: 4 mins, Cook Time: 15 mins, Serving: 1

Ingredients

- 3 organic or free-range eggplant

- 1 tsp turmeric fresh grated

- 1 tsp seeds chia

- 2 tbsp cream or coconut milk organic

- sea salt one Pinch

- 2 tsp olive oil cold pressed

- 100 g leaves of baby spinach

- 1 tbsp Pesto Super Greens

Instructions

1. Whisk together the eggplant, sea salt, chia turmeric, & coconut milk till it's blended.

2. Place some olive oil in a saucepan and heat it to medium-low temperature.

3. Sauté the spinach for around 30 secs, or unless it has wilted.

4. Turn off the heat and remove your spinach from the saucepan.

5. Heat some olive oil in a 20cm small pan, on medium heat

6. In a large bowl, whisk together the eggplants and water until smooth.

7. Fold in some wilted spinach after adding the other ingredients.

8. Add greens pesto to this pan, then serve & enjoy right away.

Nutritional Facts: Cal: 249, Carb 36 g, Fat: 5 g, Protein: 8 g

4. Chai-Spiced Buckwheat & Chia Seed Porridge

Prep Time: 10 Mins, Cook Time: 15 Mins, Serving: 6-8

Ingredients

- 1 cup rinsed buckwheat

- ½ cup of oats

- 2 tbsp seeds chia

- 2 cups cow's, soy, almond, milk

- 2 cups of water

- 2 each pear & apple, skin on grated

- 1 tsp each ginger ground & cinnamon

- ½ tsp each cardamom & nutmeg ground

- 2 tbsp butternut

- 1 tsp extract vanilla

- 2 tbsp of honey

- **Instructions**

1. Put together the buckwheat, oats, & cold water in a small bowl. Separate the chia seeds from the rest of the ingredients and mix them with milk in another dish. Overnight, soak both bowls over the bench.

2. Finely filter and then thoroughly rinse the buckwheat & oats.

3. Then add the remaining milk, buckwheat, oatmeal, water, grated pear & apple, nut butter, spices, vanilla & honey to your medium pot. Stir well to combine. Cook for approximately 30 mins at a low temperature, often stirring, until thick and creamy. If necessary, add extra water or milk to maintain a squishy consistency. Serve in dishes with your preferred garnishes.

Nutritional Facts: Cal: 328, Carb 49 g, Fat: 12 g, Protein: 17 g

5. Steel Cut Oats with Kefir and Berries

Prep time: 10 mins, cook time: 20 mins, Serving: 4

Ingredients

For oats:

- 1 cup oats steel cut
- 3 cups of water
- salt a pinch

For topping:

- Frozen or fresh berries/fruit
- A handful of almonds sliced, hemp seeds, pepitas, or another seed/nut
- Unsweetened kefir, store-bought or homemade
- Maple syrup drizzle
- Coconut sugar sprinkling

Instructions

1. A small pot filled with oats should be heated to a boil at medium-high heat. Leave for 2-3 mins of toasting, regularly turning or tossing the pan.

2. Bring the bring to a boil & then add the other ingredients. Allow to simmer for around 25 mins, or unless oats are soft to your preference. Reduce heat if necessary.

3. Assemble your parfait by mixing yogurt with kefir & adding fresh fruit, nuts/seeds, & sugar to taste.

Nutritional Facts: Cal: 308, Carb 31 g, Fat: 9 g, Protein: 7 g

6. The Breakfast Omwich

Prep: 30 mins, Prep Time: 20 Mins, cook time: 25 mins, Serving: 3

Ingredients

- 3 bacon slices
- 3 lightly beaten eggplants
- ½ cup Cheddar cheese grated
- 1 pinch of salt & black pepper ground
- 2 slices chopped ham cooked
- ¼ cup onion finely chopped
- 1 tbsp chopped fresh chives
- ¼ cup fresh mushrooms chopped
- ¼ cup of green finely chopped bell pepper
- 1 tsp jalapeno pepper finely chopped
- 2 drops pepper sauce hot
- 4 slices of toasted bread
- 2 tbsp of mayonnaise

Instructions

1. Cook the bacon until it is crisp and browned in a pan over medium heat. Drain over paper towels after removing the ice from the machine. Crumble the cooled cake when it's cold enough to handle.

2. In a mixing dish, combine the eggplants & Cheddar cheese unless well-combined. Use salt & pepper to taste. Place a skillet on medium heat and add the eggplant mix. Layer the ham, bacon, onion, green pepper, chives, mushrooms, or pepper sauce on top of the eggplants after the bottoms are set. If you want it spicy, add some pepper sauce to the mix. Add the last 1/4 cup of Cheddar cheese on top. Fold in some eggplant mixture on filling ingredients just until they're combined. Cook till cheese melts & the bottom becomes brown, then flip and cook till golden on the other side. Take off the heat and let sit for 10 mins.

3. Place two pieces of bread on each dish, and if preferred, top each with a thin layer of mayonnaise. Place one-half of the eggplant's mixture on each slice of bread. Cut every omelet in two & serve immediately after topping with the leftover bread.

Nutritional Facts: Cal: 660, Carb 30 g, Fat: 48 g, Protein: 26 g

7. Breakfast Potatoes

Prep Time: 20 mins, cook time: 30 mins, Serving: 4

Ingredients

- 4 medium russet potatoes
- 1 onion, roughly chopped
- 2 tbsp olive oil

- 1 tbsp ground cumin

- 1 pinch salt and ground black pepper to taste

- ¼ cup butter, cut into 4 pieces

- 4 slices bacon, chopped

- ¼ cup shredded sharp Cheddar cheese

Instructions

1. Set the oven at 350 degrees Fahrenheit and prepare the dish (175 deg C).

2. Place potatoes & onion in a bowl, then slice into fourths. Toss in the cumin, oil, salt, olive & pepper to taste. Refrigerate the dish until ready to bake, then cover using plastic wrap & put in the oven.

3. On your baking sheet, spread the potato-onion mix evenly. 1 slice of butter in every corner of your potatoes should be placed on top of the butter.

4. Bake for 30 mins till potatoes are fork-tender within the preheated oven.

5. To make the bacon brown uniformly, cook on medium heat for 10-12 mins while the potatoes continue baking, turning often. Drain on a platter lined with paper towels.

6. Serve the potatoes hot from the oven on a serving plate. Add Cheddar & bacon to taste.

Nutritional Facts: Cal: 515, Carb 44 g, Fat: 33 g, Protein: 10 g

8. Quinoa bread

Prep time: 10 mins, Cook time: 20 min, Servings: 4

Ingredients

- Whole uncooked quinoa seed 300 g

- Water 1/2 cup

- Grapeseed oil 60 ml (¼ cup)

- Sea salt 1/2 tsp

- key lime 1/2, juiced

Instructions

- Soak the quinoa in lots of water in the fridge (overnight) (cold). Preheat the oven to 320 degrees Fahrenheit (160 degrees Celsius).

- Rinse the quinoa in a colander after draining it. Ensure that all of the water has been removed from the sieve. In a food processor, combine the quinoa and water.

- Combine half a cup of water, sea salt, grape seed oil, and key lime juice in a mixing bowl.

- In a food processor, combine all ingredients (3 mins). The bread mixture will be consistent, with some quinoa remaining in the mix.

- Spoon the loaf pan lined with baking paper on all sides and the base.

- Bake for 1.5 hours, or until hard to the touch, and springs back when pressed with fingers.

- After removing it from the oven, let it cool for half an hour in the pan; after removing the cake, cool on a rack. The bread will be crunchy on the exterior and moist in the center.

- Allow it to cool fully before eating.

Nutrition Facts Per Serving: fat 13 g, Carb 5 g, cal 152, protein 17 g

9. Camp Breakfast

Prep Time: 15 mins, Cook Time: 26 mins, Serving: 2

Ingredients

- 6 slices cut crosswise bacon
- 1 tbsp of olive oil
- 3 cubed white potatoes
- to taste salt & black pepper ground
- 1 chopped onion
- 4 beaten eggplants

Instructions

1. On medium heat, cook & toss the bacon until it's crispy, approximately 5 mins. Discard most of the oil after transferring to a plate lined with paper towels to drain.

2. Add olive oil to the skillet and heat on medium heat. Cook & stir the potatoes for approximately 10 mins, or until they are browned & crispy.

3. Potatoes should be combined with onion and cooked until transparent, approximately five mins. Stir in the bacon & cook for another 1-2 mins, often stirring, to ensure it is cooked through.

4. Cook & whisk the eggs until they are set, 5-6 mins, over the potato mixture.

Nutritional Facts: Cal: 562, Carb 49 g, Fat: 49 g, Protein: 28 g

10. Breakfast Strata

Prep Time: 20 mins, Cook Time: 1 hr 15 mins, Serving: 8

Ingredients

- 1 lb casings removed the sausage
- 2 cups fresh mushrooms sliced
- 8 beaten eggplants
- 10 cups day-old bread cubed
- 3 cups milk whole
- 2 cups Cheddar cheese shredded
- 1 & ½ cups Forest ham cubed Black
- 1 package frozen-thawed & drained, chopped spinach
- 2 tbsp flour all-purpose
- 2 tbsp powder mustard
- 1 tsp salt
- 3 tsp melted butter
- 2 tsp basil dried

Instructions

1. Grease a 9-by-13-inch casserole dish generously.
2. Cook & stir sausage for approximately 10 mins, until crumbled and well-browned in a large pan on medium heat. Place the cooked sausage in the casserole dish that has been set aside.
3. Cook & stir mushrooms for 5-10 mins until liquid is released & they are gently browned in this skillet on medium heat; drain.

4. Put everything in a big bowl except the sausage & mix well. Then pour on the mixture. Refrigerate, covered, for at least 2 hr or perhaps overnight, the casserole dish.

5. Preheat the oven to 350°F (175 deg C).

6. Bake within the preheated oven for 60-70 mins, till a knife stabbed into the middle comes out clean.

Nutritional Facts: Cal: 600, Carb 32 g, Fat: 37 g, Protein: 34 g

11. Superfood Breakfast

Cook time: 5 mins, Prep Time: 5 mins, Serving: 1

Ingredients

- 1 cup plain yogurt nonfat
- ¼ cup of blueberries
- 2 tbsp goji berries dried
- 1 tbsp flax seed ground
- 1 tbsp walnuts ground
- 1 tbsp almonds ground
- 1 tsp cocoa powder unsweetened
- ½ tsp cinnamon ground
- ½ tsp of honey

Instructions

1. To make the yogurt granola, combine yogurt with goji berries, blueberries, and flaxseed in a dish.

Nutritional Facts: Cal: 347, Carb 43 g, Fat: 11 g, Protein: 20 g

12. Breakfast Pasta

Prep time: 10 mins, cook time: 30 mins, Serving: 4

Ingredients

- ½ package of spaghetti
- 3 tbsp divided olive oil
- 4 beaten eggplants
- ½ diced onion
- ¼ cup baby Bella mushrooms chopped
- ¼ cup peas frozen
- ¼ cup carrots shredded
- ½ cup Parmesan cheese freshly grated
- salt & black pepper ground

Instructions

1. Bring a big saucepan to a boil with a little salt in it. Cook the spaghetti in a large pot of boiling water for 12 mins, or until al dente but still firm to a biting. Drain.

2. Cook and whisk the eggplants within heated oil until they are set & scrambled, approximately 5 mins. Heat some oil inside a pan on medium heat.

3. In a different pan, heat the oil on medium-high heat & cook the mushrooms, peas, onion, & carrots for approximately 10 mins, or until the onion gets brown. Toss the spaghetti with the onion mixture. Mix in the eggplant swell. Toss the spaghetti mixture with the Parmesan, salt, & pepper that you've just added.

Nutritional Facts: Cal: 412, Carb 42 g, Fat: 17 g, Protein: 18 g

13. Breakfast Wellington

Prep Time: 15 mins, Cook Time: 45 mins, Serving: 12

Ingredients

- 1 lb sausage ground

- 1 package thawed broccoli chopped frozen

- ½ cup cream sour

- 1 cup Cheddar cheese shredded

- 2 cans roll refrigerated dough crescent

- 1 white eggplant

Instructions

1. Set the oven to 325°F (165 deg C).

2. In a large, shallow skillet: Add sausage and brown on both sides, about 10 mins total. Cook until uniformly browned on both sides over moderate flame. Drain, crush and store in a separate container for later use.

3. Cook frozen broccoli for 5 mins in a saucepan over medium heat, covered.

4. Then combine all of the ingredients in a big bowl and stir well.

5. A flattened, one crescent roll packet should be placed in a baking dish. Add the broccoli mixture on top. Then, using a serrated knife, close the edges of the leftover crescent rolls around the filling. Top with beaten eggplant white and let dry.

6. Cook for around 20 mins till golden brown into a preheated oven.

Nutritional Facts: Cal: 362, Carb 17 g, Fat: 26 g, Protein: 11 g

14. Breakfast Kolaches

Prep Time: 30 mins, Cook Time: 15 mins, Serving: 18

Ingredients

- 1 cup milk warm

- 1 lightly beaten eggplants

- 3 cups flour bread

- ½ tbsp of salt

- 3 tbsp butter

- ½ cup sugar white

- 3 tsp yeast bread machine

Instructions

1. Place eggplant, salt, butter, bread flour, and sugar in the sequence recommended by its manufacturer within the bread machine. Press the Start button after selecting the Dough cycle.

2. Set the oven to 375°F (190 deg C). Prepare a baking sheet by lightly greasing it.

3. Punch down the dough, then divide it equally into 36 pieces on a floured board. Form the pieces in balls by rolling them in sugar. Place the balls on the lined baking sheet in a thin layer approximately 2" apart. Allow for a 15–20-min rise time for the balls.

4. Form depressions in the center of the balls by flattening them out. One sausage, hash browns and cheese should be placed in each crepe. Fill each crepe with the ingredients listed above.

5. Bake for 15-18 mins, or unless the top is just beginning to brown.

Nutritional Facts: Cal: 176, Carb 8 g, Fat: 13 g, Protein: 8.6 g

15. Breakfast Chilaquiles

Prep Time: 10 mins, Cook Time: 10 mins, Serving: 2

Ingredients

- 1 & ½ tsp olive oil

- 3 tortillas corn

- 5 eggplants

- to taste salt & black pepper ground

- ¼ cup Cheddar cheese shredded

- ½ can sauce enchilada

Instructions

1. In a skillet, heat the olive oil on medium heat. Cook & toss the tortilla squares for approximately 5 mins until they are crispy.

2. Combine the eggplant, salt, & pepper, then whisk until well combined. On top of it, crumble in some Cheddar cheese.

3. Fill a pan halfway with the eggplants & cheese mixture; heat for approximately 5 mins, or unless the eggplants are set. On top of it, pour enchilada sauce.

Nutritional Facts: Cal: 373, Carb 19.3 g,

Fat: 23.4 g, Protein: 22.1 g

Lunch Recipes

1. Lunch Biscuits

Prep Time: 10 mins, Cook Time: 20 mins, Serving: 8

Ingredients

- 2 tbsp sauce pizza

- 1 cup Cheddar cheese shredded

- cooking spray

- ½ cup ham chopped

- 1 can biscuit dough refrigerated buttermilk

Instructions

1. Set the oven to 375°F (190 deg C). Grease eight muffin tins generously.

2. In a large bowl, combine ham, Cheddar cheese, & scallions, fold into biscuit pieces. Lightly combine the pizza sauce & the other ingredients. Fill prepared muffin tins about two-thirds of the way with the batter.

3. Puff & brown your biscuits inside a preheated oven for around 20 mins. Allow cooling in the muffin cups for 10 mins before removing.

Nutritional Facts: Cal: 185, Carb 16 g, Fat: 10 g, Protein: 7.1 g

2. "Heart-Friendly" Salsa

Prep time: 25 mins, Cook time: 35 min, Servings: 4

Ingredients

- Blueberries 1 Cup

- Strawberries 5

- Sea Salt 1 Pinch

- Grape Seed Oil 2 Tbsp.

- Red Onion 1/4

- Green Bell Pepper Chopped 1/3 Cup

- Chopped Avocado 1/2

- Two Key Limes Juice

Instructions

- In a blender food or processor, combine blueberries, key lime juice, onion, key lime zest, strawberries, and green bell pepper and beat roughly 5-6 times.

- If desired, season with cayenne pepper and sea salt.

- Scrape the salsa and fold in the avocado (chopped) in a mixing bowl.

Nutrition Facts Per Serving: fat 18.7 g, Carb 38 g, cal 359, protein 27.2 g

3. Foolproof Spinach & Feta Frittata

Prep Time: 10 mins, Cook Time: 15 mins, Serving: 2

Ingredients

- 2 tsp of olive oil
- 1 peeled & finely sliced small brown onion
- 4 eggplants
- 1 tsp garlic
- 251 g of baby spinach
- ½ cup feta cheese crumbled
- to taste Salt & pepper

Instructions

1. Prepare your grill by turning the burners to medium-high.

2. Melt the butter in a medium-sized frying pan with a nonstick coating which you can place underneath the grill to crisp the outside.

3. Cook the onion, occasionally stirring until it softens and browns. Toss in the spinach for a few seconds to let it wilt. Allow the dish to cool completely after removing it from the heat source.

4. In a separate dish, whisk the eggplant until light and fluffy. After the spinach & onion have been allowed to cool, stir in the feta cheese. Add salt and pepper to your liking.

5. Reheat your frying pan over medium heat before adding the eggplant. Make sure the eggplants don't set too quickly by stirring gradually until you see them. Take it off the heat and serve the frittata while it's still warm.

6. The frittata should be brown & cooked after 2-3 mins underneath the grill.

7. To release the frittata, place the plate on the pan & swiftly but gently flip it over. Serve cold or hot and accompanied with a crunchy salad on the side.

Nutritional Facts: Cal: 436, Carb 35 g, Fat: 15 g, Protein: 6 g

4. Lentil, Beetroot and Hazelnut Salad with a Ginger Dressing

Prep Time: 10 mins, Cook Time: 10 mins, Serving: 2

Ingredients

- 1 cup rinsed Puy lentils

- 2 & 3/4 cup water filtered

- salt Sea

- 3 beetroots cooked

- 2 finely sliced spring onions

- 2 tbsp roughly chopped hazelnuts

- roughly chopped fresh mint A handful

- roughly chopped fresh parsley A handful

Instructions

1. Lentils should be cooked for 15–20 mins until tender but still have a bit of bite to them, so place them in a pot, cover with some water, bring to the boil, then decrease heat & simmer till the liquid has gone & the lentils aren't mushy.

2. Make a big bowl and set it aside to chill after the lentils are done cooking.

3. After the lentil dish has calmed down, beets, spring onions, hazelnuts, and herbs may be added.

4. The dressing is as simple as combining the ginger with the mustard, oil, & vinegar in a dish and blending until smooth.

5. Serve the salad with a drizzle of the dressing on top.

Nutritional Facts: Cal: 516, Carb 55 g, Fat: 19 g, Protein: 12 g

5 Quick and Easy Quinoa Orange Salad

Prep Time: 10 Mins, Cook Time: 20 Mins, Serving: 1

Ingredients

- 1 cup cooled cooked quinoa

- 2 supreme small oranges

- 1 finely chopped celery rib

- 20 g chopped Brazil nuts

- 1 sliced green onion

- ¼ cup finely chopped fresh parsley

Instructions

1. Cut fresh oranges in supreme on a bowl to prevent any juice from dripping out. After you've completed all your supreme, ensure to squeeze out all of the remaining "membranes" of juice.

2. Use a small food processor to puree the juice. Blend in the remaining dressing ingredients until well-combined.

3. Prepare a medium-sized mixing basin, then add orange supreme. Cut them up into bite-sized pieces & stir well. Stir in the dressing & the other ingredients unless everything is well-combined.

4. Keep inside your fridge until prepared to serve or serve immediately.

Nutritional Facts: Cal: 337, Carb 38 g, Fat: 21 g, Protein: 14 g

6. Mom's Grilled Sauerkraut Avocado Sandwich

Prep Time: 10 Mins, Cook Time: 12 Mins, Serving: 2

Ingredients

- 1 cup of sauerkraut
- 8 slices bread pumpernickel
- 1 avocado
- buttery spread vegan
- 1 cup of hummus

Instructions

1. Prepare by preheating the oven to 450°F (230 deg C). Cut the 8 pieces of bread in half, butter each side, & arrange four on the baking sheet. Distribute the hummus among the four pieces of bread. Place the sauerkraut on top of hummus on every slice and serve immediately.

2. Slices of avocado should be placed on top of the sauerkraut. Repeat with leftover 4 pieces of bread on avocado slices. For golden brown & crispy sandwiches, bake within the oven for around 6-8 mins, flipping the sandwiches halfway through. Bake for another 6 mins.

Nutritional Facts: Cal: 319, Carb 39 g, Fat: 14 g, Protein: 10 g

7. Zucchini for Lunch

Prep Time: 2 mins, Cook Time: 10 mins, Serving: 3

Ingredients

- 1 tbsp oil vegetable

- 1 large, cubed zucchini

- 1 chopped medium onion

- 1 seeded & chopped bell pepper

- 2 beaten eggplants

- ½ cup tomato sauce canned

Instructions

1. Medium-high heat oil into a big skillet. Cook & stir the zucchini until it is tender, about 5 mins. Cook the onion & bell pepper for 5 mins or until soft. Pour the eggplants into the middle of the pan after creating a path there with a spatula. To scramble the eggs, heat them in a saucepan while stirring constantly. Stir the tomato sauce into the cooked eggplants until well-coated. Ideally, serve this dish when it's still warm.

Nutritional Facts: Cal: 142, Carb 11.6 g, Fat: 8.3 g, Protein: 6.8 g

8 Easy and Yummiest Kulfi Recipe

Prep Time: 10 mins, Cook Time:8 hr, Serving: 12

Ingredients

- 2 cans milk evaporated

- 2 cans table cream canned

- 1 can condensed milk sweetened

- 2 white bread slices

- ¼ tsp cardamom ground

- 12 almonds blanched

Instructions

1. To make breadcrumbs in a pudding, combine cream, evaporated milk, & condensed milk into a blender. In a food processor or blender, combine cardamom & almonds; process for 3-4 mins, until smooth. Frozen 8 hr or overnight in a glass dish. Cut into squares & serve.

Nutritional Facts: Cal: 256, Carb 22.5 g, Fat: 15.6 g, Protein: 4.8 g

9. Basil Pesto "Zoodles."

Prep time: 30 mins, Cook time: 40 min, Servings: 6

Ingredients

- Zucchini 1 lb.

- Grapeseed oil 1 tbsp.

- Avocado 1

- Basil Leaves 1/2 Cup

- Walnuts 1/4 Cup

- Olive Oil 1/4 Cup

- Sea Salt 1/2 Tsp

- Cayenne Pepper 1/4 Tsp.

- Cherry Tomatoes 1 Cup

- One Key Lime Juice

Instructions

- Begin by sauteing the zucchini noodles in grapeseed oil until they are slightly mushy but still crisp.

- Combine the remaining ingredients in a blender or food processor and pulse until a creamy, thick mixture forms.

- Stir in the drained pasta and toss well to incorporate. If the sauce seems too thick, thin it up with a little water.

- Serve with cherry tomato halves and "cheese" dissected coconut on top (shredded).

Nutrition Facts Per Serving: fat 14 g, Carb 52 g, cal 377, protein 21 g

10. Creamy Beet Detox Soup

Prep time: 15 mins, Cook time: 15 min, Servings: 8

Ingredients

- Avocado 1

- Medium beet 1/2

- Carrots 2 chopped

- 1 garlic clove

- Raw apple cider 2 tbsp. (Vinegar)

- Cayenne pinch

- Sea salt ½ tsp

- Water or coconut water 1 cup

- 1 lemon juice

- Pepper as per your taste

Instructions

- In a blender, combine all the ingredients and mix until smooth and creamy.

Nutrition Facts Per Serving: fat 12 g, Carb 47.9 g, cal 298.9, protein 13 g

11. School Lunch Bagel Sandwich

Prep Time: 10 mins, cook time: 5 mins, Serving: 1

Ingredients

- 1 tbsp cream cheese herb & garlic flavored

- 1 split & toasted multigrain bagel

- 2 thin Cheddar cheese slices

- 2 slices pickled dill

- ¼ cup carrot shredded

- 1 lettuce leaf

Instructions

1. A toasted bagel should be spread with cream cheese. One ½ of your bagel should be topped with Swiss cheese & the other half should be topped with carrots & lettuce. Wrap your sandwich in plastic wrap/ Al foil after cutting it in two. Pack your sandwich inside an ice-filled lunch bag.

Nutritional Facts: Cal: 476, Carb 66.8 g, Fat: 16 g, Protein: 20 g

---

12. Lunch Box Pita Pockets

Prep Time: 10 mins, Cook Time: 10 mins, Serving: 1

Ingredients

- ½ cup chopped deli ham

- ½ cup lettuce shredded

- ¼ cup carrot shredded

- ¼ cup dressing Ranch

- 1 pita cut bread round

Instructions

1. Salad & carrot may be combined in a zip-top bag. Fill a small, airtight container with Ranch dressing and store it in the refrigerator. Place your pita bread inside a zip-top bag and seal the bag. Lunch is ready when you have the ham and ranch dressing combination packed in your lunch bag with 1 spoon.

2. Pita pockets may be assembled by spooning this ham mix into every pita half & sprinkling with Ranch dressing before eating.

3. Mozzarella cheese, chopped pepperoni, & pizza sauce are just a few possible combinations. Other options include chopped bacon, chopped tomato, shredded lettuce, & ranch dressing.

Nutritional Facts: Cal: 559, Carb 36.6 g, Fat: 37.7 g, Protein: 17.1 g

13. Bum's Lunch

Prep Time: 15 mins, Cook Time: 45 mins, Serving: 4

Ingredients

- 4 steaks cube

- 4 thinly sliced medium potatoes

- 1 thinly sliced large onion

- 4 tsp of margarine

- to taste salt & pepper

Instructions

1. Set the oven at 350 deg Fahrenheit and prepare the dish (175 deg C).

2. Prepare Al foil in four squares. Each sheet of foil should have a cube steak on it. Season the steaks with pepper and salt after spreading them with margarine. Add a diced potato & a couple of onion rings over the top of every steak before serving. Taste and adjust the seasoning, adding more salt or pepper if necessary. Seal the package by folding the foil over the food & tying it shut. The baking sheet is a good place to put the packets.

3. Cook the potatoes for 45 minutes in your preheated oven unless they are fork-tender. Open with caution since hot steam would be emitted if you do not.

Nutritional Facts: Cal: 326, Carb 40.8 g, Fat: 10 g, Protein: 18.7 g

14. Cheese Quesadilla Lunch

Prep time: 10 mins, Cook Time: 10 mins, Serving: 1

Ingredients

- ¼ cup salsa prepared

- 1 & ½ tbsp shredded Cheddar cheese reduced fat

- 1 tbsp Parmesan cheese shredded

- 1 tbsp drained & rinsed black beans canned

- ½ tbsp fresh cilantro chopped

- 2 tortillas whole-wheat

- ½ tsp melted butter

- 1 tbsp guacamole prepared

- 1 tbsp bell peppers red chopped

Instructions

1. Set the oven to 375°F (190 degrees C).

2. In a bowl, combine salsa, cheeses (Cheddar, Parmesan, & black beans), black beans, & cilantro. Spread a thin layer of the salsa mixture over the middle of each tortilla. Top with remaining tortilla and serve. Brush the top of the quesadilla with butter once it's been placed on the baking sheet & is ready to serve.

3. Bake for 9-12 mins unless the cheese melt & the top begins to brown. Use the pizza cutter to cut the quesadilla into thin slices. Serve with guacamole & bell pepper on the side.

Nutritional Facts: Cal: 259, Carb 48.6 g, Fat: 6.9 g, Protein: 13.1 g

15. Orange Lunch Box Cookies

Prep Time: 10 mins, Cook Time: 20, Serving: 6

Ingredients

- ¾ cups of butter
- 1 cup brown sugar packed
- 1 egg, large
- 1 tbsp zest orange
- 1 tsp extract vanilla
- 2 cups of sifted flour all-purpose
- 3 tsp powder baking
- ½ tsp salt
- ½ cup of walnuts chopped
- ¼ cup sugar white

Instructions

1. Margarine/butter should be creamed, and brown sugar should be added gradually. Grate the orange peel and mix in the vanilla extract once you've added the unbeaten egg and other ingredients. Beat the hell out of it.

2. Bake for 30 mins at 350 degrees. Add sifted flour & salt to the mixture. Make sure everything is well-combined. Refrigerate dough for at least an hr or until it becomes firm.

3. Preheat the oven to 350°F (175 deg C).

4. Nuts & granulated sugar should be combined. Make walnut-sized dough balls by rolling them out to a thin disc. Sprinkle sugar & nut mixture over flattened cookies in a cookie pan that has been buttered. Ten mins in the oven should be enough. Keep cool in a drawer or on a rack. Be sure to store it in an airtight container or pan.

Nutritional Facts: Cal: 607, Carb 78.5 g, Fat: 30.6 g, Protein: 7.1 g

16. Creamy Detox Spinach Soup

Prep time: 5 mins, Cook time: 10 min, Servings: 6

Ingredients

- Water 1 cup

- Spinach 1 ½ cups

- Ginger root 1 tsp

- Sea salt ½ tsp

- Dairy-free milk ½ cup

- Cumin dash

- Avocado 1

- Stalk celery 1

- 1 garlic clove

-

Instructions

- In a blender, combine all ingredients and mix until smooth and creamy.

Nutrition Facts Per Serving: fat 14 g, Carb 39.7 g, cal 375, protein 26

17. Creamy Detox Carrot Soup

Prep time: 10 mins, Cook time: 5 min, Servings: 3

Ingredients

- Avocado 1

- Carrots chopped 2

- Milk/coconut water ¾ cup (dairy-free)

- Onion ½

- Lemon juice ¼

- Cayenne pepper 1 pinch

- Ginger 1 tsp

- Cinnamon ½ tsp

- Tahini/sun butter 3 tbsp.

Instructions

- To get a creamy, smooth texture, combine all ingredients in a blender and mix until smooth.

Nutrition Facts Per Serving: fat 12 g, Carb 34 g, cal 231, protein 17 g

18. Superfood Salad

Prep time: 15 mins, Cook time: 30 min, Servings: 8

Ingredients

- Red quinoa 1 cup (cooked)
- Beans 1/2 cup (sprouted adzuki)
- Kimchi 1/2 cup (diced)
- Avocado 1 sliced
- Broccoli head 1/2
- Carrot 1 (thin strips)
- Fresh kales leaves1 cup
- Radishes 3 (thin slices)
- Pomegranate 1 (only seeds)
- Flax seeds 2 tsp (crushed)
- Hulled hemp 1 tbsp.
- Lemon juice 1/2
- Salt (pink Himalayan) 1/4 tsp
- Flaxseed oil 2 tsp

Instructions

- In a mixing bowl, combine all ingredients and sprinkle with flaxseed oil and lemon juice before serving.

Nutrition Facts Per Serving: fat 12 g, Carb 33 g, cal 272, protein 9 g

19. Lunch Box Zucchini Slice

Prep Time: 20 mins, Cook Time: 30 mins, Serving: 8

Ingredients

- 1 tsp oil vegetable
- 3 grated zucchinis
- 6 lightly beaten eggplants
- 1 finely chopped large onion
- 1 cup flour self-rising
- 1 grated carrot
- 3 thin diced bacon slices
- 1 ½ cups Cheddar cheese shredded
- to taste salt & black pepper ground

Instructions

1. Set the oven at 350 degrees Fahrenheit and prepare the dish (175 deg C). Prepare a 6x10-inch baking dish by smearing oil all over the surface.

2. Stir in a bowl all the ingredients except for the bacon & cheese, then season with pepper and salt. Pour the mixture into the baking dish that has been previously prepared.

3. Bake for 30-40 mins, depending on how firm you want your pudding. Slice once it's been given time to cool.

Nutritional Facts: Cal: 227, Carb 16.3 g, Fat: 12.3 g, Protein: 13 g

20. Basic Keto Summer Salad

Prep Time: 15 mins, Cook Time: 15 mins, Serving: 1

Ingredients

- 2 cups mixed spring
- ¾ cup halved cherry tomatoes
- ⅔ cup cucumber chopped
- ½ cup salami sliced
- ⅓ cup red onion chopped
- ⅓ cup cheese blue
- ⅓ cup vinegar red wine
- 1 tbsp olive oil extra-virgin

Instructions

1. Serve with a side of blue cheese & a dish of spring mix. Toss your salad with the vinegar-oil dressing, which has been whisked together within a mixing bowl.

Nutritional Facts: Cal: 693, Carb 27.8 g, Fat: 52.3 g, Protein: 32.3 g

21. Raw Energy Balls

Prep time: 15 mins, Cook time: 25 min, Servings: 6

Ingredients

- Blueberries 1/2 Cup

- Shredded Coconut 2 Cups

- Walnuts 1/2 Cup

- Dried Dates 1/2 Cup

- Date Sugar 1 Tsp.

- Agave Syrup 1 Tbsp.

- Sea Salt 1 Pinch

Instructions

- First, crush the walnuts or Brazil nuts in a high-powered blender or food processor to make the powder.

- Combine the blueberries, dry dates, and date sugar in a mixing bowl. Slowly drizzle in the agave syrup until you have a paste.

- Refrigerate the mixture for 30 mins to 2 hours.

- Coat them into 1 tbsp. Balls, and then roll them in extra coconut if desired (shredded). It will keep for about a week in the fridge and three months in the freezer.

Nutrition Facts Per Serving: fat 8 g, Carb 38.4 g, cal 356, protein 19 g

22. Shrimp and White Bean Salad

Prep Time: 15 mins, Cook Time: 4 hr, Serving: 6

Ingredients

- 1 package thawed & tails removed cooked shrimp frozen

- 1 can drain & rinse cannellini beans

- 1 cup coarsely chopped cherry tomatoes

- ½ cup red onion diced

- 2 tbsp olive oil

- 2 tbsp vinegar red wine

- 1 tbsp seasoning Italian

- 1 tsp salt garlic

- 6 cups greens salad

Instructions

1. Put in a dish and combine shrimp, cherry tomatoes, cannellini beans, & red onion.

2. The shrimp mixture is coated with olive oil, vinegar, red wine, Italian spice, & garlic salt in a medium bowl. Wrap the bowl into a plastic cover and refrigerate it for at least four hr to overnight.

3. Upon serving, scatter the shrimp mixture over the leaves in a salad dish.

Nutritional Facts: Cal: 190, Carb 14.2 g, Fat: 5.9 g, Protein: 19.7 g

23. Asian Cucumber Salad

Prep time: 20 mins, Cook time: 35 min, Servings: 6

Ingredients

- Key lime juice 3 tbs.

- Sesame oil 1 tbs.

- date sugar 1/2 tsp

- Sea salt 1/4 tsp

- grated ginger 1 tbs.

- Sesame seeds 1 tbs.

- Granulated seaweed 1 tbs.

Instructions

- To make the salad, toss all of the ingredients together and serve.

Nutrition Facts Per Serving: fat 17.3 g, Carb 31 g, cal 269, protein 15 g

24. Herb-Crusted Cauliflower Steaks with Beans and Tomatoes

Prep Time: 15 min, Cook Time: 30 Mins, Serving: 2

Ingredients

- 1 large cauliflower head

- ½ cup divided olive oil

- 2 tsp divided kosher salt

- 1 tsp of freshly ground divided black pepper

- 8 oz trimmed green beans

- 3 finely chopped garlic cloves

- ¾ tsp lemon zest finely grated

- ⅓ cup parsley chopped

- ⅓ cup of panko

- ¼ cup Parmesan freshly grated

- 1 can rinse, drained white beans

- 1 cup halved red or golden cherry tomatoes

- 3 tbsp of mayonnaise

- 1 tsp mustard Dijon

-

Instructions

1. Preheat the oven at 425 degrees Fahrenheit and place racks in the center and top thirds of the oven. The core of the cauliflower should be left intact. Remove the leaves and cut the end of the stalk. On the work surface, place the cauliflower core-side down. Cut the middle of the cauliflower into two 1-inch "steaks" with a big knife; save the rest for later use.

2. Bake the cauliflower in the center of a preheated oven to 400°F. Brush 1 Tbsp. Oil on both sides; 14 tsp. Salt & 14 tsp. Pepper over both sides. Roast on the center rack for 30 mins, tossing halfway through to brown and soften the cauliflower.

3. Meanwhile, stir green beans using oil, salt, & pepper. Roast in the oven for around 15 mins or unless the green beans start to blister.

4. Whisk salt and pepper in a large bowl unless smooth. Stir in garlic, parsley, lemon zest, and the leftover oil. Place half mixture in a small bowl and stir to combine. Mix in the panko & Parmesan using your hands once you've added them to the first bowl. Toss in the white beans & tomatoes from the first dish with the dressing from the second. In a bowl, combine mayonnaise & mustard.

5. Take the baking sheets out of the oven. Spread the cauliflower with the mayonnaise mix. Over the cauliflower, evenly distribute the

6. 1/2 cup panko mixture. Toss the white bean mixture with the green bean mixture on the baking sheet. After 5–7 mins, remove the baking pans from the oven & continue roasting the white beans till crisp and the panko coating has browned.

7. Distribute the cauliflower, white beans, green beans, & tomatoes

8. among serving bowls & plates to taste. Add some fresh parsley on the top if desired.

Nutritional Facts: Cal: 231, Carb 12 g, Fat: 5 g, Protein: 7.3 g

Dinner Recipes

1. Homemade Vegetarian Chili

Prep Time: 20 mins, Cook Time: 40 mins, Serving: 4-6

Ingredients

- 2 tbsp olive oil extra-virgin
- 1 medium chopped red onion
- 1 large, chopped bell pepper red
- 2 chopped medium carrots
- 2 ribs celery chopped
- ½ tsp divided salt
- 4 minced or pressed cloves garlic
- 2 tbsp powder chili
- 2 tsp cumin ground
- 1 & ½ tsp paprika smoked
- 1 tsp oregano dried
- 1 can large, diced tomatoes
- 2 cans rinsed & drained black beans
- 1 can rinse & drain pinto beans
- 2 cups of vegetable water or broth
- 1 leaf bay
- 2 tbsp fresh cilantro chopped
- 1-2 tsp vinegar sherry

Instructions

1. Warm your olive oil to a shimmering state in an oven or heavy saucepan over medium heat. Chopped carrots and onions should be added along with the 1/4 tsp of salt. Cook, occasionally stirring, for 7 to 10 mins or until the veggies are soft and the onion has become translucent. Make a spice blend by combining all dry ingredients except the oregano. About 1 min of cooking time until aromatic with continual stirring is required. Add black beans, vegetable broth, pinto beans, & bay leaf to the chopped tomatoes & their liquids. Allow the mixture to get to your simmer once you've given it a good stir. Cook for another 30 mins, stirring regularly and lowering the heat as needed to keep the mixture at a slow simmer.

2. Discard your bay leaf after removing the chili from heat. Transfer the chili to your blender, including some liquid, for the greatest texture & taste. Pour the combined mix back in the saucepan, cover tightly with a lid, & process until smooth (careful of hot steam!). Alternately, puree the chili until it has a thicker, chili-like appearance using a potato masher. Stir in the chopped cilantro & vinegar to taste before serving. Add additional salt as desired. Serve with your favorite toppings once you've divided the mixture into separate bowls.

Nutritional Facts: Cal: 398, Carb 29.2 g, Fat: 16.2 g, Protein: 8.3 g

2. Joseph's Best Easy Bacon Recipe

Prep Time: 5 mins, Cook Time: 15 mins, Serving: 6

Ingredients

- 1 package bacon thick cut

Instructions

1. Lay down two sheets of Al foil on a baking sheet, being careful to cover the whole surface area of the pan. Bake bacon on a parchment-lined baking sheet in a single layer, about 1/2 inch apart. Placing the pan in a cold oven can help it cook faster. Set the oven to 425°F (220 deg C). 14 mins is the recommended cooking time for bacon. Place roasted bacon on dishes lined with paper towels. Allow 5 mins of cooling time so the bacon can crisp up.

Nutritional Facts: Cal: 134, Carb 0.4 g, Fat: 10.4 g, Protein: 9.2 g

3. Curried Shrimp & Vegetables Recipe

Prep Time: 10 mins, Cook Time: 15 mins, Serving: 4

Ingredients

- 3 Tbsp coconut oil butter
- 1 sliced onion
- 1 cup milk coconut
- 1-3 tsp powder curry
- 1 lb tails removed shrimp
- 1 bag frozen veggies or frozen cauliflower

Instructions

1. The sliced onion should be added to melted butter/oil in a pan. Make sure the onion is tender but not mushy by sautéing it unless it is. While all of this is going on, start steaming some veggies. Stir in coconut milk, curry powder and other seasonings once the onion has softened.

2. Cook for a couple of mins to let the flavors come together. Cook the thawed shrimp for about 5 mins, or until they are done. Steamed vegetables with butter & a salad dressing go well with this dish.

Nutritional Facts: Cal: 332, Carb 11.2 g, Fat: 22.7 g, Protein: 23.9 g

4. Sleep-time drink

Prep time: 20 mins, Cook time: 25 min, Servings: 2

Ingredients

- Cooked quinoa 1/4 cup
- Amaranth greens 2 cups
- Burro banana 1
- Cherries 1/4 cup
- Agave syrup

Instructions

- Begin by making the tea for the Sleepy Time drink (Dr. Sebi).
- Allow time for it to cool.
- Combine all ingredients in a blender and serve.

Nutrition Facts Per Serving: fat 16.4 g, Carb 31 g, cal 281, protein 21.5 g

5. Seven-veg stir-fry 20

Prep time: 30 mins, Cook time: 15 min, Servings: 1

Ingredients

- Thai rice noodles 250g pack
- Groundnut oil 1-2 tbsp.
- Red pepper 1, deseeded & cut in thumb-length strips
- 2.5cm fresh root ginger (1in) piece, peeled & cut into slivers
- Baby sweetcorn 8, halved lengthways
- Carrots 2 medium, peeled & cut in batons
- Asparagus tips 8
- Mini sugar-snap peas/mange tout 3½ oz.
- Sweet chili dipping sauce 4tbsp/hoisin sauce
- Optional red chili 1, deseeded & chopped finely
- Pak choi 2 heads, quartered lengthways
- Fresh beansprouts 100g/150g pack
- Spring onions 4-6, trimmed & thinly sliced
- Mint & coriander leaves, chopped roughly
- To serve Soy sauce

Instructions

- Add the noodles to a big bowl and pour ample boiling water to cover them. Leave it for 5 mins. As you cook vegetables in a large frying pan or hot wok, add oil (1 tbsp.) and stir the ginger and red pepper for half a minute. Add the asparagus, carrots, and sweetcorn and for a min, stir-fry, add the mange tout or sugar snaps and simmer for one more min.

- Mix in the hoisin or chili dipping sauce and 4 tbsp water, add the pack Choi, red chili, spring onions, and beansprouts, and cook for a few minutes.

- Toss it with coriander and mint. For seasoning, serve topped with soy sauce and stir-fried vegetables.

Nutrition Facts Per Serving: fat 14.6 g, Carb 37.2 g, cal 382, protein 21.3 g

6. Roasted cauliflower, fennel, and ginger soup

Prep Time: 3 mins, Cook Time: 20 Mins, Serving: 3

Ingredients

- 1 quartered red onion

- 4 cloves garlic

- ½ large cauliflower head

- 2 chopped & cored fennel bulbs

- 500 g choice stock

- 3 tbs hummus

- 1 Tbsp Gut Blend Golden

- 1 tsp leaves sage

- fennel seeds pinch

- 2 tbs tamari wheat-free

- 2 tbs lemon fresh

- 1 peeled knob ginger

Instructions

1. Preheat the oven to 200°C. Toss the fennel & the cauliflower together with the red onion over a baking sheet. Bake till crispy, about 30 to 35 mins.

2. Take out of the oven & combine with the other ingredients inside a blender. Blend until smooth and fluffy, about a min or two. Place on the stovetop inside a heavy-bottomed pot. Permit flavors to blend over low heat for the duration of the cooking process.

3. Add salt and pepper to your liking. Serve warm, after allowing it to cool somewhat. Fennel fronds may be used to decorate.

Nutritional Facts: Cal: 357, Carb 45 g, Fat: 21 g, Protein: 15.4 g

7. Sleep-time drink

Prep time: 20 mins, Cook time: 25 min, Servings: 2

Ingredients

- Cooked quinoa 1/4 cup

- Amaranth greens 2 cups

- Burro banana 1

- Cherries 1/4 cup

- Agave syrup

Instructions

- Begin by making the tea for the Sleepy Time drink (Dr. Sebi).

- Allow time for it to cool.

- Combine all ingredients in a blender and serve.

Nutrition Facts Per Serving: fat 16.4 g, Carb 31 g, cal 281, protein 21.5 g

---

8. Quick Orecchiette Pasta with Kale Pesto

Prep time: 15 mins, Cook time: 25 min, Servings: 2

Ingredients

- Fresh Kale 1 bunch roughly chopped

- Bunch fresh basil 1 small

- Sage leaves 2 fresh

- Garlic cloves 3

- Toasted pine nuts 1 cup

- Extra virgin olive oil 2 tbsp.

- Dijon mustard 1 tsp

- Red chili flakes 1/2 tsp

- Lemon 1/2 juice

- Sea salt Pinch

- Orecchiette pasta 1/2 box 2 cups

- Fresh lemon juice, toasted pine nuts, red chili flakes to garnish:

Instructions

- Put the new herbs, garlic, lemon juice, and olive oil in a mixing bowl and pulse several times to form a mash.

- Add the chili flakes, Dijon, pine nuts, and salt, and pulse a few times to combine.

- Place the mixture in a jar with a cover.

- Cook the orecchiette according to the Instructions.

- Transfer to a large mixing dish and stir in 3 tbsp fresh pesto until fully combined.

- Divide the mixture into bowls. Season with red chili flakes and toasted pine nuts, then sprinkle with fresh lemon juice and olive oil before serving.

Nutrition Facts Per Serving: fat 21 g, Carb 49 g, cal 399, protein 26 g

9. Easy Kielbasa Skillet Dinner

Prep Time: 20 mins, Cook Time: 35 mins, Serving: 4

Ingredients

- ½ chopped onion

- 1 package sliced kielbasa sausage

- cooking spray

- ½ cut head broccoli

- 3 peeled & sliced potatoes

- salt & black pepper ground

Instructions

1. Lightly grease an 8-inch skillet & place it on medium heat. Sauté the onion within the oil in a large pan over medium heat for 5 mins, occasionally stirring until transparent. Stir in kielbasa and cook for an additional 5 mins, turning regularly, until the sausage is gently browned.

2. Season sausages mix with pepper and salt, then stir in broccoli & potatoes. Allow to cook, uncovered, for approximately 15 mins, or until broccoli is tender. Cook, occasionally stirring, for an additional 10-15 mins, or till veggies are soft when pierced with a fork.

Nutritional Facts: Cal: 492, Carb 34.9 g, Fat: 31.3 g, Protein: 18.3 g

10 Easy Dinner Hash

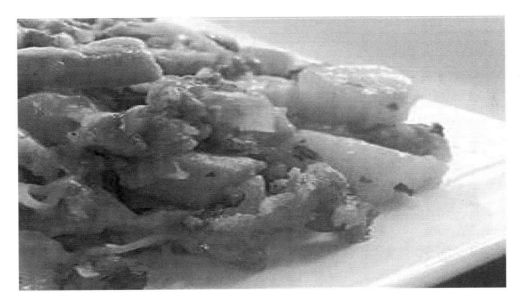

Prep Time: 15 mins, Cook Time: 20 mins, Serving: 2

Ingredients

- 1 tbsp oil vegetable

- 8 oz sausage bulk Italian

- 1 peeled & diced potato

- ¼ chopped onion

- 1 cup mixed vegetables frozen

- to taste salt & pepper

- ¼ cup Cheddar cheese shredded

Instructions

1. In a skillet, warm the vegetable oil on medium heat. Add the sausage & cook for 5 mins, occasionally stirring, till crumbled and a still little pink in the center. Add the potato & onion, then mix well. The potatoes should be soft and gently browned by this point, perhaps 10-15 mins more.

2. Stir in all mixed veggies when your potatoes are ready, and heat through. Use salt & pepper to your liking and adjust the seasoning, if necessary, before serving, top with some Cheddar cheese.

Nutritional Facts: Cal: 622, Carb 27.2 g, Fat: 46.9 g, Protein: 23.4 g

12. Parmesan Crusted Dinner Rolls

Prep Time: 15 mins, Cook Time: 20 mins, Serving: 12

Ingredients

- 1 cup Parmesan cheese grated

- 1 loaf frozen-thawed bread dough

- ½ cup melted salted butter

Instructions

1. Make a small bowl and add the Parmesan cheese to it.

2. Next, cut every piece of bread dough in three more for 36.

3. Melt the butter & then roll every piece into a ball.

4. Gently push the greased dough ball in the shaved Parmesan cheese with your fingers.

5. Put three of the coated balls in each of the muffin tins prepared.

6. Keep covered with a cloth & let to rise till doubled in size, 5-7 hr, based on the ambient temperature (80-95 deg F).

7. Set 375 degrees F in the oven (190 degrees C).

8. Cook for 20-25 mins till golden brown within the preheated oven.

Nutritional Facts: Cal: 203, Carb 18.4 g, Fat: 11.1 g, Protein: 6.4 g

13. Zucchini Noodles with Cilantro Pesto

Prep time: 20 mins, Cook time: 35 min, Servings: 6

Ingredients

- For the cilantro pesto:

- Cilantro 1 bunch

- 1/2 lemon Juice of

- Cloves garlic minced 2-3

- Pine nuts 1/4 cup

- Salt 1/2 tsp

- For the zucchini noodles:

- Large zucchini 2

- Heirloom tomatoes 2 sliced

- Salt

Instructions

- Combine the cilantro, lemon juice, garlic, olive oil, pine nuts, and salt in a food processor. Pulse until the ingredients are coarsely minced. If necessary, transfer to a mortar and pestle to finely ground and release flavors.

- Cut the zucchini ends to make all sides flat. Connect it to a spiralizer with the Julienne blade (thin) to produce noodles.

- Heat the olive oil in a pan over medium heat. Toss in the zucchini noodles and heirloom tomatoes, cut. Heat and turn with a salt sprinkle until the zoodles are soft but still hold their form, about 3-5 mins.

- Serve the cilantro pesto over the heirloom tomatoes and zucchini noodles until heated.

Nutrition Facts Per Serving: fat 12.9 g, Carb 31 g, cal 295, protein 17 g

14. Roast tomato and orange soup recipe

Prep time: 15 mins, Cook time: 35 min, Servings: 2

Ingredients

- Tomatoes 900g

- Chopped 2 garlic cloves

- Olive oil 4 tbsp.

- Diced onions 2

- Carrots peeled/scrubbed 2

- Diced celery sticks 1

- Hot vegetable stock 560ml

- Orange juice 100ml

- For serving the zest of 1 small orange

- (optional) Edible flowers

Instructions

- Preheat the oven to 160°C/180°C (gas/fan mark 4)

- Arrange the tomatoes and sprinkle with chopped garlic on a large baking pan. Season with salt and black pepper and 2 tbsp olive oil. When the oven is hot, Place the tomatoes in the oven and roast for 45 mins, stirring halfway through.

- After stirring the tomatoes, heat the remaining olive oil in a large, deep skillet and sauté the carrots, onions, and celery for 20 mins on low heat. Toss in the garlic and roasted tomatoes. Return to the pan and add the orange juice and stock to the tank, giving it a brief stir.

- Bring the soup to a simmer for 1-2 mins, then remove it from the heat and allow it to cool before liquidizing. To the skillet, Return the soup to the pot and taste for seasoning, adding more salt and black pepper if necessary. If you're going to serve it right away, make sure it's hot enough.

- If you're serving the soup cold, let it cool completely before transferring it to a large container and chilling it for a few hours.

- Serve garnished with orange zest and edible flowers such as borage or nasturtium.

Nutrition Facts Per Serving: fat 13 g, Carb 37 g, cal 361, protein 24 g

15. Vegetarian Pizza with Autumn Toppings

Prep time: 15 mins, Cook time: 10 min, Servings: 2

Ingredients

For the Crust

- Whole wheat flour 2/3 cups

- Dried yeast 1/2 tbsp.

- Brown sugar 2 tsp

- Extra virgin olive oil 1 tbsp.

- Warm water 2/3 cups

- Salt 1/2 tsp

- Cornmeal 1 tbsp.

- For the Toppings

- Roasted pumpkin cubes 1 cup

- Roasted bell pepper 2 cuts in thin stripes

- Lacinato kale leaves 5 roughly chopped

- Goat cheese crumbled 1/2 cup

- Lightly toasted walnuts 1/4 cup

- Pickled onion rings 5-6

- Honey 1 tsp

- Tomato passata 2 tbsp.

- Minced garlic cloves 2

- Extra virgin olive oil 2 tsp

- Pomegranate 1/2 seeds

Instructions

- In a mixing dish, combine the water, sugar, and yeast; set aside for ten minutes to dissolve the yeast.

- Combine the salt and flour in a large mixing bowl, pour over the yeast mixture, add the olive oil, and stir with a fork.

- Transfer the mixture to a floured area and knead for about five mins, or until an elastic dough forms. If the mixture is too moist, add another tbsp of flour.

- Place the dough in a dish, cover with a towel, and set aside to rise for thirty mins at room temperature.

- Preheat the oven to 200 degrees Celsius.

- Form the pizza dough into an oval or thin circle.

- Place the pizza dough on a cookie sheet lined with bakery release paper and sprinkle with cornmeal.

- Toss the minced kale, goat cheese, garlic, and pumpkin into the pizza dough, then thinly spread the passata on top.

- Bake for fifteen mins, then remove from oven and season with walnuts, pickled onion, and pomegranate seeds.

- Drizzle with honey and serve warm.

Nutrition Facts Per Serving: fat 17 g, Carb 36 g, cal 294, protein 21 g

16. One-pot zucchini mushroom pasta

Prep time: 20 mins, Cook time: 25 min, Servings: 8

Ingredients

- Spaghetti 1 lb

- Cremini mushrooms 1 lb thin sliced

- Thinly sliced 2 zucchini & quartered

- Sprigs thyme 2

- Cayenne pepper & Sea salt to taste

Instructions

- In a large stockpot or Dutch oven over medium-high heat, combine the pasta, mushrooms, zucchini, and thyme, along with 4 1/2 cups water; season to taste with sea salt and cayenne pepper.

- Bring to a boil; decrease the heat to low and continue to cook, uncovered, for 8-10 mins or until liquid is reduced.

- Add homemade walnut milk to the mix.

- It's practical to serve and drink.

Nutrition Facts Per Serving: fat 12.1 g, Carb 41 g, cal 327, protein 26 g

1. Fruit Race Cars for Kids

Prep Time: 10 mins, Cook Time: 0 mins, Serving: 2

Ingredients

- Apples
- Knife
- Cutting board
- Seedless grapes
- Rounded toothpicks

Instructions

1. Prepare your fruit by washing and prepping it. Rinse with some water and use a solution of bicarbonate soda & salt to remove waxy residue. Repeat the procedure of rinsing and drying.

2. Cut the apple into thirds, then thirds again. Each apple provides enough food for 12 people.

3. Both core & seeds may be easily removed from apple wedges by making a clean, straight cut around the fruit.

4. Transversely insert two toothpicks into the apple wedge, one in every flat end.

5. Feed the toothpicks with four full grapes. The automobile would be more stable if the grapes were larger.

Nutritional Facts: Cal: 318, Carb 42.5 g, Fat: 11.2 g, Protein: 10.3 g

2. Matcha Green Smoothie Bowl

Prep Time: 5 Mins, Cook Time: 5 Mins, Serving: 2

Ingredients

- 2 ripe bananas peeled, sliced & frozen
- ¼ cup ripe pineapple chopped
- ¾ - 1 cup coconut milk light
- 2 tsp tea powder matcha green
- 1 cup heaping kale or organic spinach

Instructions

1. A high-speed blender combines pineapple, banana slices, reduced coconut milk, matcha powder, & spinach. Blend till creamy & smooth.

2. Just enough coconut milk to aid in the blending is all you need to add. This smoothie should fall somewhere in the middle between scoopable & drinkable.

3. Add additional banana to make it sweeter, more matcha to give the green tea taste more intensity, or a splash of coconut milk to make it creamier if desired. Add additional pineapple if you want it tart/tangy.

4. Divide into two serving dishes, top with selected toppings. Chia seeds, Fresh raspberries, & coconut flake were my choice ingredients. Bananas would be a great addition as a garnish.

5. Fresh is best, but leftovers store nicely in the fridge for almost 24 hr if well wrapped.

Nutritional Facts: Cal: 175, Carb 34.8 g, Fat: 5 g, Protein: 2.9 g

3. Free-Spirited Nachos

Prep Time: 10 Mins, Cook Time: 15 Mins, Serving: 3-4

Ingredients

- 2 diced tomatoes
- 1 diced cucumber

Nachos chips

- 100 g meal almond
- 1 large egg organic
- 1 tsp of turmeric
- ¼ tsp cumin
- ¼ tsp coriander
- 1 tsp orange zest grated
- 1 tsp sea salt Celtic

Instructions

1. Preheat your oven to 180°C before making the chips.

2. Mix all chip ingredients using a wooden spoon in a big bowl to make a dough.

3. Place your dough between two sheets of baking paper over the clean work area. The dough should be rolled out to a thickness of 2 mm (1/16").

4. Move the dough & bottom baking paper on a baking pan, then remove a top sheet of the baking paper. Score your dough deeply, each 3 cm (11/4") with a paring blade to make squares. Repeat the process in the other way.

5. 12 mins in the oven are the recommended cooking time.

6. Before separating them, let them cool completely.

7. Add the additional ingredients over top of Nachos chips over a cutting board to construct nachos.

8. The remaining chips may be stored inside an airtight jar in the refrigerator for three days.

Nutritional Facts: Cal: 258, Carb 24.5 g, Fat: 12.3 g, Protein: 7.3 g

4. Cashew Sour Cream

Prep Time: 10 Mins, Cook Time: 10 Mins, Serving: 1

Ingredients

- 155 g cashews raw, unsalted
- 2 tsp vinegar apple cider
- 2 tbsp lemon juice freshly squeezed
- 1 & 1/2 tsp yeast flakes nutritional
- ¼ tsp sea salt Celtic

Instruction

1. Allow the cashews to soak into filtered water for at least two hr before using. Drain and rinse thoroughly.

2. All components should be placed in your food processor using filtered water & blended until completely smooth.

3. If the mixture is too thick, add a bit of additional filtered water.

4. This will stay in the refrigerator for 2 to 3 days, sealed.

Nutritional Facts: Cal: 237, Carb 40.3 g, Fat: 9.2 g, Protein: 4.5 g

5. Creamy Avocado Dressing

Prep Time: 10 Mins, Cook Time: 5 Mins, Serving: 4

Ingredients

- 1 peeled & stone removed avocado

- 1 tsp heaped powder cumin

- large lime juice 1

- 1 tsp zest lime

- sea salt Celtic big pinch

- 1 tbsp cold-pressed olive oil extra virgin

Instructions

1. Using a food processor, puree all components except olive oil till smooth, adding 2 tsp filtered water if needed.

2. Add some olive oil into a stream while the machine runs until the required creaminess is achieved.

3. It will keep inside the refrigerator for 3-4 days, sealed.

Nutritional Facts: Cal: 128, Carb 14.5 g, Fat: 2.5 g, Protein: 1.03 g

6 Coconut-Chia Pudding-in-a-Jar

Prep Time: 10 mins, Cook Time: 5 Mins, Serving: 1

Ingredients

- One can make coconut milk light

- 3 tbsp seeds chia

- 3 tbsp syrup pure maple

- ½ cup pineapple chunks fresh

- 2 medium peeled & sliced kiwis

- ¼ cup of raspberries

- 2 tbsp chopped roasted almonds

Instruction

1. Combine chia seeds, coconut milk, & maple syrup. Four 8 oz glass jars should hold the whole mixture. To thicken in a pudding, chill the mix, covered, overnight to enable all seeds to fatten up.

2. Over the top of your pudding, put the kiwi, raspberries, pineapple, & almonds. Freeze for

   almost one day, covered with a lid.

Nutritional Facts: Cal: 221, Carb 28.5 g, Fat: 19.2 g, Protein: 15.3g

7. Ultimate Power Balls

Prep Time: 10 Min, Cook Time: 30 Min, Serving: 25

Ingredients

- ½ cup millet puffed
- 1 cup puffed rice or puffed Kamut
- ½ cup dried plums diced
- 1/3 cup chocolate chips semisweet
- ¼ cup seeds sesame
- 1/3 cup butter sunflower
- ½ cup of honey
- ¾ cup coconut shredded unsweetened

Instruction

1. Toss the puffed millet & puffed Kamut / rice in a wide bowl. Add dried plums, chocolate chips, & sesame seeds to the mixture.

2. Add both sunflower butter & honey and mix well after each addition. You should be covered with goo! Freeze the bowl for around 30 mins after covering it with plastic wrap.

3. To prepare the coconut, put it in a shallow basin and mix it with the sugar. Form the mixture into 1" (2.5cm) balls using your hands after scooping it up with a tbsp. Place the coconut-coated balls in a jar and set them aside. In the zip-top refrigerator bag, keep these power balls for almost 1 month within the refrigerator or up to 1 week within the freezer.

Nutritional Facts: Cal: 291, Carb 54.1 g, Fat: 12.4 g, Protein: 16.3 g

BOOk 20:

Drinks and Smoothies

1. The Anti-Inflammation Smoothie!

Prep Time: 5 mins, Cook Time: 0 Min, Serving: 2

Ingredients

- 1 inch grated fresh ginger
- 1 inch grated fresh turmeric
- baby spinach A handful
- watercress A handful
- 1 avocado small
- ½ bell pepper
- a handful of coriander or parsley flat-leaf
- 1 cup water coconut
- Cayenne a Big pinch
- salt a Pinch

Instructions

1. Blend the roots, avocado, & coconut water in a food processor until smooth.
2. This should be blended to produce a foundation.
3. After that, combine all of the ingredients in a blender & process until smooth.

Nutritional Facts: Cal: 125, Carb 19.5 g, Fat: 4.1 g, Protein: 1.3 g

---

2. Alkaline Smoothie

Prep Time: 3 mins, Cook Time: 2 mins, Serving: 2

Ingredients

- 1 cup milk almond
- 1 cup cubed watermelon
- 5 frozen strawberries
- 1/2 banana small
- 1 fresh spinach handful
- 1 tsp seeds chia
- 1 cup of ice

Instructions

1. Blend your ingredients in the order given on the container.
2. Blend the ingredients in the blender till smooth and well-combined.

3. To avoid a dark smoothie, combine greens with chia seeds, banana, ice, & almond milk before blending.

4. Almond milk & ice are added to a watermelon strawberry mixture.

5. Combine the smoothies within the same glass & serve immediately.

Nutritional Facts: Cal: 81, Carb 14 g, Fat: 2 g, Protein: 2 g

- 1 cup of water

Instructions

1. Wash kale and spinach, peel lemon (leaving pith on), then toss all ingredients into the blender and blend until smooth for about 1 min.

Nutritional Facts: Cal: 58, Carb 14.5 g, Fat: 3 g, Protein: 2.3 g

3. Energizing Alkaline Smoothie with Kale, Mango and Spinach

Prep Time: 5 mins, Cook Time: 1 min, Serving: 1

Ingredients

- 2 kale leaf's large dinosaur
- spinach 1 handful
- 1 banana, fresh
- 1/2 cup chopped mango frozen
- 3 thumb-sized ginger knobs
- 1 lemon, fresh

4 Minty Alkaline Kiwi Green Smoothie

Prep Time: 10 mins, Cook Time: 5 Mins, Serving: 2

Ingredients

- 1 kiwi, spooned out sliced half & flesh
- 1 peeled & sliced green apple
- 1/2 diced English cucumber
- 1 cup tightly packed spinach
- a fresh mint small handful

- 2 tsp honey pure
- 1 tsp zest lemon
- 1/2 medium lemon juice
- 1 banana, fresh
- ¼ cup of water
- optional 1 tbsp coconut oil raw

Instructions

1. Blend all ingredients till smooth & creamy in your blender for around 30-60 seconds. If you'd want it sweeter, you can always add additional honey or a banana.

Nutritional Facts: Cal: 238, Carb 45.7 g, Fat: 7.7 g, Protein: 2.8 g

---

5. Alkaline Green Smoothie

Prep Time: 10 mins, Cook Time: 20 Mins, Serving: 2

Ingredients

- 2Kiwi Fruit
- 180 g Honeydew Melon
- 1Cucumber
- 10 g Ginger Root Fresh
- 120 g Baby Spinach Fresh
- 2 tsp Lemon Juice
- 200 mL Coconut Water or water

Instructions

1. Cucumber, melon, & ginger root should all be peeled.

2. Please put them in your food processor with spinach & lemon juice, then process until smooth.

3. Blend all ingredients in a high-speed blender until they are completely smooth.

4. If a smoothie is still too thick for your liking, add a little more water (coconut water).

5. When you're done, pour your green juice into glasses & serve immediately.

6. Store in the refrigerator for almost 2 days in jars/bottles with tight-fitting caps.

Nutritional Facts: Cal: 152, Carb 41.5 g, Fat: 23 g, Protein: 1.2 g

Nutritional Facts: Cal: 244, Carb 34.5 g, Fat: 12.1 g, Protein: 4.2 g

7. Alkaline Blueberry Banana Smoothie Recipe

Prep Time: 5 mins, Cook Time: 5 mins, Serving: 1

Ingredients

- 1 banana ripe
- ½ cup of blueberries
- 1 tsp greens powder alkaline
- 1/2 tbsp flaxseed ground
- 1/2 tbsp seeds hemp
- 1/2 cup of ice
- 1/2 cup of milk
- 1/2 cup of water

Instructions

1. Blend the banana, hemp seeds, blueberries, flaxseed, greens powder, & ice with the milk and water until smooth.

6   Super   Alkaline   Cherry Smoothie

Prep Time: 15 mins, Cook Time: 15 mins, Serving: 1

Ingredients

- 1 & ½ cup almond milk
- 1 cup fresh cherries, seeded
- 1 cup stems removed fresh kale
- 1 peeled kiwi
- 2 tbsp cashews raw
- ½ chopped fresh beet

Instructions

1. In a high-powered blender, combine all ingredients until well-combined.

2. Blend the ingredients in a blender until they are completely smooth.

2. Put the lid on and mix for 1-2 mins, or until the ingredients are completely processed & smooth. Blueberries & hemp seeds may be used as a garnish if desired. Enjoy!

Nutritional Facts: Cal: 68, Carb 16.5 g, Fat: 12.1 g, Protein: 2.3 g

8 Alkaline Lime Smoothie

Prep Time: 5 Min, Cook Time: 10 Mins, Serving: 2

Ingredients

- 3/4 cup water or coconut water
- 1 tbsp coconut creamed or ½ cup young coconut, Thai
- 2 cups baby spinach firmly packed
- 1 pitted & peeled medium avocado
- 1/2 chopped medium cucumber
- 2 tbsp lime zest finely grated
- 2 peeled & halved limes
- 20 drops liquid stevia alcohol-free
- natural salt a Pinch
- 1 & 1/2 cups of ice cubes

Instructions

1. Then, blend at high for 30-60 secs, unless the mixture is smooth & creamy again.

Nutritional Facts: Cal: 78, Carb 17.2 g, Fat: 10.2 g, Protein: 4.3 g9. Alkalizing Apple Green Smoothie

Prep Time: 5 Mins, Cook Time: 10 Mins, Serving: 2

Ingredients

- 1 Apple Large
- 3 spinach Handfuls
- ½ cup of water
- ¼ cup of pumpkin seeds

Instructions

1. Cover the pumpkin seeds with water and let them soak overnight.
2. Remove the water from the pumpkin seeds and add the seeds to a blender.

3. Remove the core and seeds from the apple and chop it. Add it to the blender.

4. Add the spinach to the blender.

5. Blend until smooth. Add as much water as you need if you want to drink it or leave it as it is and eat with a spoon.

Nutritional Facts: Cal: 84, Carb 12.8 g, Fat: 9.2 g, Protein: 5.3 g10 Cucumber & Kale Smoothie

Prep Time: 5 mins, Cook Time: 5 mins, Serving: 1

Ingredients

- 1 cucumber, fresh
- curly kale A handful
- 1 tsp honey clear
- 1 cup of coconut water
- lemon juice 1 squeeze
- 1 tsp juice ginger

Instructions

1. Cucumbers should be cleaned and rinsed before use. Please put it in a blender once you've cut it up into little bits.

2. Rinse & add fresh Kale leaves to the cucumber mixture once they have been well washed.

3. Blend everything else in your blender.

4. To make a well-mixed smoothie, blend & process your cucumber mixture until it is smooth.

5. The smoothie will have a much more refreshing flavor and boost alkaline content with lemon juice.

6. Adding the juice from half a ginger root provides the smoothie with a subtle kick of spice.

Nutritional Facts: Cal: 441, Carb 89 g, Fat: 4 g, Protein: 16 g

11. Triple Berry Smoothie

Prep Time: 5 mins, Cook Time: 6 mins, Serving: 2

Ingredients

- 1 cup water alkaline
- 1 cup blueberries frozen
- 1/2 cup raspberries frozen
- 1/2 cup blackberries frozen
- 1/2 cup quinoa cooked
- 2 halved & pitted Medjool dates

Instructions

1. High-speed blender: Combine the water & all of the berries (blackberries, blueberries, raspberries, etc.) with the quinoa & dates. High-speed blending for around 60 secs, or till smooth.

2. Prepare the drink and serve it right away.

Nutritional Facts: Cal: 312, Carb 34.4 g, Fat: 18.1 g, Protein: 23.7 g

Prep Time: 5 mins, Cook Time: 5 mins, Serving: 2

Ingredients

- 2 cups Water Filtered
- 4 cups of Spinach
- 1 Banana Frozen
- 2 cups Pineapple Frozen
- 1 Tbs Ginger Fresh
- ½ freshly squeezed Lemon

Instructions

1. Blend all greens & water till smooth in a blender.

2. Add the pineapple, ginger, banana, & lemon juices to the mixture and stir to combine. Make sure everything is well-combined.

3. The flavor is at its peak as soon as the ingredients are blended.

Nutritional Facts: Cal: 298, Carb 39.3 g, Fat: 18.1 g, Protein: 24.2 g

12 Morning Pineapple Ginger Green Smoothie

13. Alkaline Electric Burro Banana Smoothie

Prep Time: 5 Mins, Cook Time: 5 Mins, Serving: 3

Ingredients

- 1 tsp of powder baobab
- 5 bananas burro
- 2 lemon peel small pieces
- mangoes Handful
- pumpkin seeds Handful
- turmeric small piece
- 250ml of water spring

Instructions

1. Place all of the ingredients in a blender jar and mix until smooth.

2. Fill the blender halfway with spring water and mix until smooth.

3. Start the blending process. Blender speeds should be progressively increased from low to high. This will prevent the blades from becoming stuck while the contents are being thoroughly combined.

4. Then, enjoy your nutrient-dense alkaline smoothie by pouring it into a glass. Enjoy.

Nutritional Facts: Cal: 288, Carb 49.5 g, Fat: 15.6 g, Protein: 27.3 g

14. Green Power Smoothie

Prep Time: 5 Mins, Cook Time: 5 Mins, Serving: 1

Ingredients

- 1/2 cup rice milk unsweetened
- 1/4 cup dairy-free yogurt unsweetened
- 1 cup kale baby
- 1 core removed & diced apple
- 2-4 cubes of ice
- 1 tbsp melted coconut oil

Instructions

1. Blend everything except the coconut oil in your blender until smooth. Add additional rice milk if necessary to combine and reach desired consistency.

2. While your blender is spinning, carefully pour in your coconut oil by opening the lid's top. Oil does not clump together as a result of this. Taste & adjust the amount of maple syrup & lemon juice as necessary.

Nutritional Facts: Cal: 278, Carb 29.5 g, Fat: 21 g, Protein: 8.3 g

1. Spinach, cilantro, & water should be blended to a smooth consistency.

2. Blend in the leftover fruits after that.

3. Prepare the dish and serve it to your guests.

Nutritional Facts: Cal: 236, Carb 38.5 g, Fat: 11.6 g, Protein: 2.3 g

15. Mango Smoothie

Prep Time: 4 Mins, Cooking Time: 5 Mins, Serving: 2

Ingredients

- 1 & ½ cups fresh spinach
- ½ cup fresh cilantro
- 1 & ½ cups of mango
- 2 cups of water
- 2 cups of pineapple
- ½ avocado

Instructions

16. Turmeric Smoothie with Berries

Prep Time: 3 mins, Cook Time: 2 mins, Serving: 2

Ingredients

- 3/4 cup almond milk unsweetened vanilla
- 2 cups spinach baby
- 1/2 cup Greek yogurt nonfat plain
- 3 tbsp rolled oats old-fashioned
- 1 & 1/2 cups berries frozen mixed

- 1/2 tsp turmeric ground

- 1/4 tsp ginger ground

- 2-3 tsp swap agave or honey

Instructions

1. Almond milk, turmeric, ginger, spinach, berries, yogurt, & 2 tbsp of honey should all be blended in a strong blender as in order mentioned.

2. Blend the ingredients in a blender until they are completely smooth. If necessary, adjust the sweetness with a taste. The spinach, almond milk, and yogurt should be blended before adding the remaining ingredients if you don't have access to a powerful blender. Take pleasure in it right now.

Nutritional Facts: Cal: 151, Carb 27 g, Fat: 2 g, Protein: 8 g

17. 5-Min Anti-Inflammatory Smoothie Recipe

Prep Time: 5 mins, Cook Time: 5 mins, Serving: 2

Ingredients

- 1 cup mixed berries frozen

- 1 banana

- some ginger fresh

- 1 juice lemon

- 1 tbsp of flaxseed plus 3 tbsp of water

- 1 cup of water

- 1 tsp cinnamon

Instructions

1. In a blender, combine all ingredients and process until completely smooth. It takes roughly 2 mins to combine everything in a high-speed blender for blending. You can begin by blending at a low speed then gradually raise it until the job is done.

Nutritional Facts: Cal: 112, Carb 24 g, Fat: 2 g, Protein: 2 g

18. Anti-Inflammatory Pineapple Smoothie

Prep Time: 12 Mins, Cook Time: 5 Mins, Serving: 3

Ingredients

- 2 cups frozen pineapple chunks
- 1 cup frozen mango cubes
- ½ cup frozen banana
- 2 tsp turmeric paste frozen
- ¾ cup yogurt Greek
- ¾ cup orange juice freshly squeezed

Instructions

1. Place the pineapple, mango, & banana in small zip-lock bags after rough chopping them. Chop the fruits and place in the freezer for 4-6 hr, or unless frozen. You should be able to freeze anything overnight.

2. Just when you're about to prepare a pineapple smoothie, squeeze some fresh orange juice.

3. Pour all of the ingredients into a high-powered blender and mix until smooth. Add a dollop of yogurt on top if desired. Set blender to "creamy" or "smooth" mode and mix until that is the desired result.

4. If necessary, you may sweeten the smoothie with honey.

5. The mixture should be poured into glasses/bowls for serving. If you like, you may top it with a few mango chunks, pineapple chunks, and banana slices. Add a few chia seeds to the mix. Serve your smoothie right away, garnished with a pineapple slice placed on its side.

Nutritional Facts: Cal: 135, Carb 14.1 g, Fat: 3.1 g, Protein: 2.2 g

19. Anti-Inflammatory Smoothie Cubes

Prep Time: 10 Mins, Cook Time: 6 Hr, Serving: 2

Ingredients

- 3 cups mango frozen or fresh
- 1 tbsp peeled & finely grated fresh turmeric
- 1/8 tsp pepper black
- ¼ to ½ cup of water
- 3 cups pineapple fresh
- 1 tbsp fresh peeled & finely grated ginger root

Instructions

Ginger Pineapple Smoothie Cubes

1. Ginger should be peeled and coarsely grated.
2. Pineapple should be peeled and chopped before serving.
3. Blend the ginger, pineapple, and other ingredients in a strong blender until smooth.
4. Fill the ice cube plate half-full of some fruit puree & freeze until firm, about 4-6 hr.

Nutritional Facts: Cal: 143, Carb 16.3 g, Fat: 3.5 g, Protein: 2.8 g

Turmeric Mango Smoothie Cubes

1. Fresh turmeric, peeled and grated to a fine powder, should be used.
2. Peel and cut mangoes into bite-size pieces. Frozen mango may also be used.
3. Then use a strong blender to purée the mango with the grated turmeric & black pepper.
4. To puree your mango, you might have to add 1-2 cups of water.
5. Fill the ice cube pan half-full of some fruit puree & freeze until firm, about 4-6 hr.

Nutritional Facts: Cal: 155, Carb 15.4 g, Fat: 5.3 g, Protein: 2 g

3. Honey & cinnamon should be added at this point. Use two glasses to collect the juices after straining.

4. Ideally, serve this dish when it's still warm.

Nutritional Facts: Cal: 117, Carb 11.8 g, Fat: 4.3 g, Protein: 2.3 g

20. Golden Milk - Miraculous Anti-Inflammation Drink

Prep Time: 4 Mins, Cook Time: 25 Mins, Serving: 2

Ingredients

- 2 cups organic   coconut unsweetened

- 1 tbsp fresh ginger peeled grated

- 1 tbsp fresh turmeric peeled grated

- 4 peppercorns black

- 2 tsp of cinnamon

- 2 tsp local honey raw

Instructions

1. Melt the butter and add the ginger, coconut milk, & turmeric.

2. Bring the mix to the simmer and then remove from the heat. Cook for 10 mins with the lid on.

21. Anti-inflammation juice

Prep Time: 2 Mins, Cook Time: 5 Mins, Serving: 6

Ingredients

- ¼ tsp of juice lemon

- ¼ tsp of ginger dry

- 1 cup of juice cranberry

- ¾ tbsp of juice orange

- ¼ tsp nutmeg

- 1 tsp of cinnamon Ceylon

Instructions

1. Add the cinnamon, nutmeg, ginger, & cranberry juice to two glasses of boiling water. Make sure everything is well-combined before setting aside for 20 mins. After that, just stir in the orange and lemon juices to complete the cocktail.

2. You may consume it right away. It will help you lose weight by increasing your metabolism & balancing your thyroid hormones. It also has a lot of vitamins, so it helps boost immunity, reduce inflammation, & keep a variety of ailments at bay.

3. This drink would also aid digestion & assist you in losing weight.

Nutritional Facts: Cal: 161, Carb 12.9 g, Fat: 12.4 g, Protein: 2.7 g

22. Anti-Inflammatory Hot Turmeric Milk

Prep Time: 5 mins, Cook Time: 5 mins, Serving: 1

Ingredients

- ¾ cup of milk

- ¾ cup of water

- 1 tbsp fresh ginger grated

- 1 tsp of honey

- 1 tsp of ghee

- ½ tsp turmeric ground

- ½ tsp cinnamon ground

- ⅛ tsp black pepper ground

Instructions

1. Place all ingredients in a wide saucepan & heat over low heat until hot but not boiling. To boil, whisk for 5-10 mins at a medium-high temperature. Turn off the heat and remove the saucepan from the stove. Serve grated ginger straight away, strained.

Nutritional Facts: Cal: 161, Carb 6.3 g, Fat: 8.1 g, Protein: 6.3 g

23. Creamy Turmeric Drink with Honey and Ginger

Prep Time: 6 mins, Cook Time: 10 mins, Serving: 1

Ingredients

- 8 oz of milk, soy milk or almond milk
- ¼ tsp turmeric
- ¼ tsp ginger
- ¼ tsp cinnamon
- to taste honey
- 5-10 drops of vanilla extract

Instructions

1. In a medium saucepan, combine all your ingredients and warm slowly while whisking continuously (about 5 mins).

Nutritional Facts: Cal: 143, Carb 12 g, Fat: 7 g, Protein: 7 g

24. Healing 3-Ingredient Turmeric Tonic

Prep Time: 2 Mins, Cook Time: 10 min, Serving: 2

Ingredients

- 1 Tbsp grated turmeric fresh
- 1 Tbsp grated ginger fresh
- 1 lemon whole
- 1-2 tsp syrup maple
- 1 cayenne pepper pinch
- 3 cups water filtered

Instructions

1. Make an infusion of turmeric, ginger, and lemon rind in a small pot with maple syrup, cayenne, & filtered water.

2. On moderate flame, bring to the boil for about 3 mins. After then, turn the heat off.

3. Divide into two mugs using a tiny strainer set over serving glasses. Enjoy. If this tonic is strong, add extra hot or warm water to dilute it.

4. The leftovers may be stored in the refrigerator for almost 2-3 days after preparation (strained). Reheat until barely warm in a microwave or over the stovetop.

Nutritional Facts: Cal: 13, Carb 1.8 g, Fat: 0 g, Protein: 0.4 g

- Using a high-speed blender or food processor, combine the coconut water & cottage cheese with kale, mango, flaxseed, banana, and sweetener (if desired).

Nutrition Facts Per Serving: fat 6 g, Carb 56 g, Cal 311, protein 15 g

25. Mango-Coconut Green Smoothie

Prep Time: 05 Mins, Cook Time: 05 Mins, Serving: 1

Ingredients

- ½ cup water coconut
- ⅓ cup cottage cheese low-fat
- 1 cup kale chopped
- 1 cup banana slices frozen
- ½ cup mango frozen
- 1 tbsp flax meal or flaxseed
- 1 to 2 tsp pure honey or maple syrup

Instructions

26. Avocado & Arugula Omelet

Prep Time: 10 Mins, Cook Time: 10 Mins, Serving: 1

Ingredients

- 2 eggplants large
- 1 tsp milk low-fat
- ⅛ tsp divided salt
- 2 tsp of extra-virgin divided olive oil
- ½ cup of arugula
- 1 tsp juice lemon
- ¼ diced avocado
- 2 tbsp plain Greek yogurt whole-milk

Instructions

- In a mixing bowl, whisk together the eggs, milk, & a sprinkle of salt. Small nonstick skillet with oil over moderate flame. Ensure that the bottom is cooked through but that the middle is still a little runny, around 1-2 mins after adding the egg mixture. Cook for a further 30 seconds on the other side, or until the omelet is set. Put it on a serving dish.

- Combine the arugula with some oil and lemon juice in a separate dish. Avocado, yogurt, arugula, and the last sprinkle of salt go on top of the omelet.

Nutrition Facts Per Serving: fat 28 g, Carb 7 g, Cal 344, protein 17 g

- 1 & ½ cups spinach baby
- 1 small, sliced banana
- 1 cup strawberries frozen
- 6 cup coconut milk unsweetened vanilla

Instructions

- Blend spinach, strawberries, banana, and your choice of milk (such as coconut) in a food processor until smooth. If required, the tamper blends at moderate speed until the mixture is completely smooth.

- Set blender to medium-high & keep going until the mixture is silky & smooth.

Nutrition Facts Per Serving: fat 4 g, Carb 39 g, Cal 183, protein 4 g

27. Spinach Smoothie

Prep Time: 10 Mins, Cook Time: 10 Mins, Serving: 1

Ingredients

28. Kale & Spinach Smoothie

Prep Time: 10 Mins, Cook Time: 10 Mins, Serving: 1

Ingredients

- 1 cup kale baby
- 1 cup spinach baby
- 5 roughly chopped dates, pitted
- 1 sliced kiwi, peeled
- 2 tbsp almond butter creamy
- 1 cup almond milk unsweetened vanilla

Instructions

- A blender is a perfect tool for mixing this healthy green smoothie. Using the tamper, if required, continue to blend at moderate speed till the mixture is completely smooth.
- Set blender to medium-high & keep going until the mixture is silky and smooth.

Nutrition Facts Per Serving: fat 21 g, Carb 51 g, Cal 419, protein 12 g

29. Artichoke Ricotta Flatbread.

Prep Time: 10 Mins, Cook Time: 10 Mins, Serving: 4

Ingredients

- ½ lb pizza dough or homemade
- 1 & ½ cups of fresh ricotta cheese whole milk
- 2 tbsp chopped fresh basil
- 1 tbsp honey
- 8 oz drained marinated artichokes
- 6 oz prosciutto torn or fresh mortadella
- 3 cups arugula fresh
- ½ cup parmesan cheese fresh shaved
- 1 tbsp chopped fresh chives
- pepper flakes crushed red
- Lemon Vinaigrette
- 1/3 cup oil
- 1 lemon juice & zest
- 2 tsp cider vinegar

Instructions

- The oven should be preheated to 450°F. Olive oil may be used to coat a big baking sheet.

- Push/roll your dough out to a very thin layer on a floured board. The dough should be transferred to a prepared baking sheet, drizzled in olive oil & gently sprinkled with salt and pepper before baking. Take out of the oven & bake for around 8 to 10 mins, or unless the crust is brown.

- A touch of pepper and salt is all that is needed to season the ricotta. Top with ricotta after taking it out of the oven. Spread out the artichokes, then add the crushed red peppers, if desired if you'd like. Mortadella or prosciutto may be added to the dish. Add arugula & shaved parmesan to the top before serving. Drizzle the chives & lemon vinaigrette over the salad just before serving.

Nutrition Facts Per Serving: fat 25 g, Carb 12 g, Cal 551, protein 32 g

30. Walnut Sage Pesto Pasta with Roasted Delicata Squash

Prep Time: 15 Mins, Cook Time: 30 Mins, Serving: 6

Ingredients

Roasted Delicata Squash:

- 2 medium scrubbed & rinsed well delicata squash

- 2 tbsp olive oil extra virgin

- salt kosher

- black pepper freshly ground

Walnut Sage Pesto:

- 1 cup parsley leaves flat-leaf

- ¾ cup walnut halves raw or toasted

- 2 to 3 garlic cloves medium

- 6 to 7 fresh sage leaves large

- ½ cup walnut oil roasted

- salt kosher

- black pepper freshly ground

For the Pasta and Serving:

- ¼ cup olive oil extra virgin roughly

- 1 lb whole fusilli or wheat penne dried

- ½ cup Parmigiano-Reggiano finely grated

Instructions

- A temperature of 425°F should be reached in the oven. Aluminum foil may be used to cover a baking sheet. Begin boiling water for the pasta at the same time.

- Slice the delicata squash in half lengthwise and remove the seeds. Take a spoon and remove the seeds. A sheet pan is ideal for preparing this dish, so slice each squash half into 12-inch-thick half-moon slices. Spread them out over the sheet pan that they don't touch each other with a generous drizzle of salt, olive oil, & pepper. Roast your squash for 20-25 mins, rotate them midway through until they are soft and caramelized, then serve.

- Make the walnut-sage pesto while the squash is roasting. In a huge food processor equipped with a blade attachment, combine your parsley leaves, garlic cloves, walnuts, & fresh sage leaves and pulse until finely chopped. Process the oil from the toasted walnuts until it is almost smooth. Add salt and pepper to taste, then transfer to a serving dish. Fresh lemon zest or juice may be added if desired.

- Paper towels may be used to line a tiny dish. Over medium-high heat in a nonstick pan, add a thin coating of olive oil (approximately 14 cups). In batches, deep-fry the sage leaves until they are crispy. Place on a dish and sprinkle with a little salt after transferring with a slotted spoon.

- The pasta should be cooked until al dente is added to boiling water after the squash is roasting. Drain the pasta and save 1 cup of the starchy cooking water. Put the pasta back in the saucepan, then add walnut-sage pesto and shredded Parmigiano-Reggiano cheese. Drizzle with a little olive oil. The pesto will liberally cover the pasta; however, the starch cooking water would help produce a creamier, more distributed sauce. Toss till the pasta is thoroughly coated within the sauce, adding a few of the conserved pasta water as required.

- Roasted Delicate squash chunks & fried sage leaves may be added to the dish. Parmigiano-Reggiano cheese should be sprinkled over the dish.

Nutrition Facts Per Serving: fat 27 g, Carb 38 g, Cal 477, protein 11 g

31. Healthy Shrimp and "Grits" (Whole30, Keto, Paleo)

Prep Time: 02 Mins, Cook Time: 10 Mins, Serving: 2

Ingredients

For Shrimp

- 1 lb peeled & deveined large shrimp
- 2-3 tbsp seasoning Cajun
- salt
- 2 tbsp butter or ghee

For Cauliflower "Grits"

- 1 bag cauliflower frozen
- 1 large, chopped clove garlic
- 2 tbsp butter ghee
- to taste salt

Instructions

- Bring a medium pot of water to the boil with a few inches of water added. Simmer the cauliflower in the steamer basket with a big clove of chopped garlic on top until it is tender. Place a lid on the pot and heat over low heat until the vegetables are cooked.

- If desired, ghee or butter may be used instead of ghee or butter in the food processor. Keep the heating water where it is! When you are close to the ideal consistency, blitz. The final consistency may be achieved by adding salt and a little amount of hot water.

- While you're doing that, prepare your shrimp. Then generously season with Cajun spice after letting it air-dry. Don't scrimp on the coating to ensure that the shrimp are completely covered. Seasoning amounts to roughly 2-4 tsp in our house. Salt your shrimp if the Cajun spice does not contain salt.

- 2 tbsp. Ghee or butter, heat over medium-high heat in a big pan, ideally cast iron. Shrimp may be added to the pan after it's healed enough and the bottom starts to turn pink, perhaps a min or two. Cook your shrimp till they become pink on the underside on the second side. Remove your deveined shrimp from the pan as soon as they are no longer transparent in the center.

- Top the cauliflower "grits" with half of the shrimp and serve. Pour this "sauce" from a cast-iron pan, including the ghee & Cajun spice, into serving dishes. Serve at once.

Nutrition Facts Per Serving: fat 19 g, Carb 13 g, Cal 554, protein 51 g

BOOK 21:

Dr. Sebi's Healing Principles:

- **Understanding the Body's Natural Balance:**

In Dr. Sebi's holistic approach to healing, the body is viewed as a complex system that naturally seeks balance and harmony. Central to this understanding is the concept of the body's innate intelligence, which continually strives to maintain equilibrium at physical, mental, and emotional levels. Dr. Sebi emphasizes that optimal health is achieved when the body's systems are in a state of balance, characterized by proper functioning and vitality. However, imbalances can occur due to various factors such as poor diet, environmental toxins, stress, and emotional disturbances. Dr. Sebi teaches that these imbalances disrupt the body's natural harmony, leading to the onset of disease and dysfunction. By understanding the body's natural balance and the factors that can disrupt it, individuals can take proactive steps to restore harmony and promote healing. Dr. Sebi's healing principles focus on addressing the root causes of imbalance, supporting the body's innate healing mechanisms, and creating conditions conducive to optimal health and well-being. Through education, lifestyle modifications, and natural therapies, individuals can align with the body's innate wisdom and unlock its inherent capacity for healing and restoration.

- **Alkaline vs. Acidic: Restoring Harmony:**

In Dr. Sebi's holistic philosophy, the balance between alkalinity and acidity in the body plays a pivotal role in maintaining optimal health. Delving into this concept reveals a fundamental understanding of the body's biochemistry and its intricate relationship with the foods we consume. Dr. Sebi teaches that the modern diet, characterized by processed foods, animal products, and sugary beverages, tends to create an acidic environment within the body. This acidic state disrupts cellular function, impairs nutrient absorption, and weakens the immune system, laying the foundation for disease to thrive. Conversely, an alkaline state supports cellular vitality, enhances detoxification processes, and fosters overall well-being. Dr. Sebi's healing principles revolve around restoring alkaline balance by emphasizing a plant-based diet rich in alkaline foods such as fruits, vegetables, nuts, and seeds. By prioritizing alkaline-forming foods and minimizing acidic foods, individuals can create an internal environment that supports health and vitality. Through education and dietary modifications, Dr. Sebi empowers individuals to reclaim their alkaline balance, paving the way for optimal health and wellness.

The Role of Nutrition in Healing: Dr. Sebi underscores the paramount importance of nutrition in facilitating the body's innate healing processes. Nutrition, according to Dr. Sebi's teachings, serves as the foundation upon which optimal health is built, influencing every aspect of cellular function and metabolic activity. Central to Dr. Sebi's approach is the recognition that the body thrives when nourished with whole, plant-based foods that are rich in essential nutrients, enzymes, and phytonutrients. These foods provide the building blocks necessary for cellular repair, regeneration, and immune function, fostering a state of vibrant health and vitality. Dr. Sebi emphasizes the consumption of foods in their natural, unprocessed state, as they retain their full spectrum of nutrients and therapeutic properties. By prioritizing plant-based nutrition and minimizing the intake of processed, refined foods, individuals can provide their bodies with the optimal fuel needed for healing and restoration. Through education and dietary guidance, Dr. Sebi empowers individuals to make informed choices that support their health goals, guiding them towards a lifestyle centered around wholesome, plant-based nutrition as a cornerstone of healing and well-being.**BOOK 21: Dr. Sebi's Healing Principles:Detoxification for Wellness:** Dr. Sebi advocates for detoxification as a crucial aspect of achieving and maintaining overall wellness. Detoxification is the process of eliminating toxins and waste products from the body, allowing it to function optimally and regain its natural balance. Dr. Sebi offers a multifaceted approach to detoxification, encompassing various methods that target different systems and organs within the body. One of the primary methods recommended by Dr. Sebi is fasting, which allows the digestive system to rest and redirects the body's energy towards repair and detoxification processes. Fasting may take various forms, including water fasting, juice fasting, or intermittent fasting, depending on individual needs and preferences. Additionally, Dr. Sebi incorporates herbal cleanses into his detoxification protocols, utilizing the therapeutic properties of specific herbs to support the body's detox pathways and enhance elimination of toxins. These herbal cleanses may include teas, tinctures, or capsules formulated with detoxifying herbs such as burdock root, dandelion, and sarsaparilla. Furthermore, Dr. Sebi emphasizes the importance of dietary modifications as part of a comprehensive detoxification plan. This involves eliminating processed foods, refined sugars, and artificial additives from the diet while increasing the consumption of whole, plant-based foods that support detoxification and nourish the body. By adopting Dr. Sebi's methods for detoxification, individuals can purify their bodies, renew their vitality, and lay the foundation for long-term wellness and disease prevention.

Holistic Approach to Wellness:

Dr. Sebi's holistic approach to wellness transcends mere physical health, recognizing that true well-being encompasses the integration of physical, mental, and spiritual aspects of health. At the core of Dr. Sebi's philosophy is the understanding that these dimensions are interconnected and influence one another profoundly. Physical health is not viewed in isolation but as part of a larger tapestry that includes mental clarity, emotional balance, and spiritual alignment. Dr. Sebi teaches that achieving optimal health requires addressing imbalances and disharmonies at all levels of being. This holistic perspective acknowledges the profound impact of mental and emotional factors on physical health, recognizing that stress, negative thought patterns, and unresolved emotions can manifest as physical symptoms and contribute to the development of disease. Likewise, spiritual well-being is considered essential for overall health, providing individuals with a sense of purpose, connection, and inner peace. Dr. Sebi's holistic approach to wellness empowers individuals to cultivate balance and harmony across all dimensions of their being, fostering a state of wholeness and vitality. Through practices such as meditation, mindfulness, and spiritual inquiry, individuals can deepen their understanding of themselves and their connection to the world around them, enhancing their overall well-being and quality of life.

Prevention Through Lifestyle Choices:

Dr. Sebi emphasizes the profound impact of lifestyle choices on overall well-being, recognizing that preventive measures are key to maintaining health and vitality. Central to Dr. Sebi's teachings is the understanding that lifestyle factors play a significant role in the development and prevention of disease. Stress management is highlighted as a crucial component of preventive care, as chronic stress can weaken the immune system, disrupt hormonal balance, and contribute to a myriad of health issues. Dr. Sebi advocates for stress-reducing practices such as meditation, deep breathing exercises, and spending time in nature to promote relaxation and emotional resilience. Additionally, regular exercise is emphasized as essential for maintaining physical health and vitality. Physical activity supports cardiovascular health, strengthens the immune system, and promotes the release of endorphins, which are natural mood enhancers. Dr. Sebi recommends incorporating a variety of activities such as walking, yoga, and strength training into one's routine to ensure a balanced approach to fitness. Adequate rest and sleep are also prioritized in Dr. Sebi's preventive care model. Sleep is recognized as a critical time for the body to repair and regenerate, supporting immune function, cognitive health, and emotional well-being. Dr. Sebi encourages individuals to prioritize sleep hygiene practices such as maintaining a regular sleep schedule, creating a relaxing bedtime routine, and creating a comfortable sleep environment. By exploring and implementing lifestyle choices such as stress management, exercise, and adequate rest, individuals can proactively safeguard their health and well-being according to Dr. Sebi's principles.

Empowering the Body's Healing Capacity:

Dr. Sebi's healing principles are deeply rooted in the belief that the body possesses an innate capacity to heal itself when given the proper support and conditions. Central to this principle is the empowerment of individuals to take an active role in their health and healing journey. Dr. Sebi teaches that healing is not a passive process but an active collaboration between the individual and their body's natural intelligence. By understanding the body's innate healing mechanisms and the factors that support or hinder them, individuals can make informed choices that facilitate the healing process. Dr. Sebi's approach emphasizes the importance of self-awareness, education, and personal responsibility in promoting health and well-being. Through education and empowerment, individuals learn to listen to their bodies, recognize signs of imbalance, and make lifestyle choices that support optimal health. Dr. Sebi's healing principles empower individuals to become active participants in their own healing journey, fostering a sense of autonomy, empowerment, and self-reliance. By taking ownership of their health and well-being, individuals can cultivate resilience, vitality, and a deeper connection to their bodies and inner wisdom.

Addressing Root Causes:

Dr. Sebi's approach to healing is distinguished by his emphasis on identifying and addressing the root causes of illness, rather than merely alleviating symptoms. Central to this principle is the recognition that symptoms are manifestations of underlying imbalances or dysfunctions within the body. Dr. Sebi teaches that conventional medicine often focuses on treating symptoms without addressing the underlying causes, leading to temporary relief but failing to achieve lasting healing. Instead, Dr. Sebi advocates for a comprehensive approach that seeks to uncover and address the root causes of illness at their source. This involves a thorough assessment of factors such as diet, lifestyle, environmental exposures, emotional stressors, and genetic predispositions that may contribute to disease development. By identifying and addressing these root causes, individuals can address the underlying imbalances that drive disease and promote true healing and restoration.

Dr. Sebi's healing principles empower individuals to become active participants in their healing journey, fostering a deeper understanding of their bodies and the factors that influence health and well-being. Through education, lifestyle modifications, and natural therapies, individuals can address root causes, support the body's innate healing mechanisms, and achieve optimal health and vitality.

Achieving Balance and Harmony:

Dr. Sebi's healing principles are centered around the fundamental concept of restoring balance and harmony to the body. According to Dr. Sebi, vibrant health and vitality can only be achieved when the body's systems are in a state of equilibrium, free from imbalance and dysfunction. Achieving balance and harmony involves addressing the underlying imbalances that disrupt the body's natural equilibrium, whether they stem from dietary factors, environmental toxins, emotional stressors, or other sources. Dr. Sebi's approach focuses on supporting the body's innate healing mechanisms and providing the necessary conditions for restoration and renewal. By adopting a holistic approach that addresses the physical, mental, and spiritual aspects of health, individuals can create an internal environment that fosters balance and vitality. Dr. Sebi's healing principles empower individuals to take proactive steps towards achieving balance and harmony in their lives, guiding them towards a state of vibrant health and well-being. Through education, lifestyle modifications, and natural therapies, individuals can align with the body's natural rhythms and unlock its inherent capacity for healing and restoration.

Integrating Mind, Body, and Spirit:

Dr. Sebi's holistic approach to healing emphasizes the interconnectedness of mind, body, and spirit in the healing process. According to Dr. Sebi, true healing occurs when these three aspects of our being are in harmony and alignment. The mind, body, and spirit are not separate entities but are deeply interconnected and influence one another profoundly. Dr. Sebi teaches that imbalances in one aspect of our being can manifest as symptoms or illness in another, highlighting the importance of addressing all dimensions of health for holistic healing to occur.

In Dr. Sebi's view, the mind plays a pivotal role in health and healing, as our thoughts and beliefs have a profound impact on our physical and emotional well-being. Negative thought patterns, stress, and emotional trauma can manifest as physical symptoms or contribute to the development of chronic illness. Therefore, cultivating a positive mindset, practicing mindfulness, and addressing emotional imbalances are essential aspects of Dr. Sebi's holistic approach to healing.

The body is regarded as a sacred vessel that houses the essence of our being, and its health is intimately connected to our overall well-being. Dr. Sebi emphasizes the importance of nourishing the body with wholesome, plant-based foods, maintaining physical activity, and supporting detoxification processes to promote optimal health. By providing the body with the nutrients it needs and creating a supportive environment for healing, individuals can optimize their physical health and vitality.

Spirituality is also considered a vital component of healing in Dr. Sebi's holistic approach. Spirituality encompasses our connection to something greater than ourselves, whether it be nature, the universe, or a higher power. Cultivating a sense of spirituality can provide individuals with a sense of purpose, meaning, and inner peace, which are essential for overall well-being.

By integrating mind, body, and spirit in the healing process, individuals can experience profound transformation and restoration on all levels of their being. Dr. Sebi's holistic approach empowers individuals to embark on a journey of self-discovery, healing, and spiritual growth, leading to a life of balance, vitality, and fulfillment.

BOOK 22: Dr. Sebi's Guide to Detoxification:

Understanding Toxins in the Body:

Dr. Sebi's guide to detoxification begins with a comprehensive exploration of the multitude of toxins that accumulate within the body. These toxins originate from various sources, including environmental pollutants, such as heavy metals, pesticides, and air pollution, which are absorbed through the air we breathe, the water we drink, and the food we eat. Additionally, processed foods laden with artificial additives, preservatives, and chemical flavorings introduce toxins into the body, overwhelming its natural detoxification pathways. Furthermore, stress, both physical and emotional, triggers the release of stress hormones, such as cortisol, which can disrupt the body's detoxification processes and contribute to toxin buildup.

Dr. Sebi emphasizes the detrimental effects of these toxins on the body's overall health and well-being. They can accumulate in tissues, organs, and cells over time, leading to a range of health issues, including inflammation, oxidative stress, hormonal imbalances, and impaired immune function. By gaining insight into the sources and effects of toxins in the body, individuals can better understand the importance of detoxification as a foundational step towards reclaiming their health.

Dr. Sebi's guide provides detailed information on how toxins affect different systems and organs within the body, highlighting their role in the development of chronic diseases and degenerative conditions. By understanding the impact of toxins on health, individuals are empowered to take proactive steps to reduce their toxic burden and support the body's natural detoxification processes. Through education, dietary modifications, and targeted detoxification protocols, individuals can embark on a journey towards optimal health and vitality by cleansing their bodies of harmful toxins and restoring balance and harmony within.

The Detoxification Process:

Dr. Sebi's guide to detoxification delves into the intricacies of the body's natural detoxification pathways and offers insights into supporting them through his recommended methods. The human body possesses sophisticated mechanisms for detoxification, primarily carried out by organs such as the liver, kidneys, lungs, skin, and lymphatic system. These organs work synergistically to neutralize and eliminate toxins from the body, ensuring its overall health and vitality.

Dr. Sebi emphasizes the importance of supporting these natural detoxification pathways to optimize their function and enhance the body's ability to eliminate toxins efficiently. One of the key methods recommended by Dr. Sebi is through dietary modifications, particularly by adopting a plant-based diet rich in alkaline foods. Alkaline foods help to alkalize the body and support the liver's detoxification processes, allowing it to efficiently metabolize and eliminate toxins.

In addition to dietary changes, Dr. Sebi advocates for herbal cleanses and supplements that specifically target detoxification pathways. These herbal remedies are carefully selected for their detoxifying properties and may include herbs such as burdock root, dandelion, milk thistle, and bladderwrack. These herbs support liver function, enhance kidney filtration, promote lymphatic drainage, and facilitate the elimination of toxins through sweat and urine.

Furthermore, Dr. Sebi emphasizes the importance of hydration in the detoxification process. Adequate water intake is essential for supporting kidney function and flushing toxins out of the body. Drinking purified water and herbal teas can help to facilitate detoxification and promote overall well-being.

Dr. Sebi's guide to detoxification provides individuals with practical strategies for supporting the body's natural detoxification pathways and enhancing its ability to eliminate toxins effectively. By adopting a holistic approach that addresses diet, herbal supplementation, hydration, and lifestyle factors, individuals can embark on a journey towards detoxification, renewal, and optimal health.

Herbal Remedies for Detoxification:

Dr. Sebi's guide to detoxification introduces readers to his carefully curated selection of detoxifying herbs and elucidates how they facilitate cleansing of the liver, kidneys, and other vital organs. Dr. Sebi's approach to detoxification centers around harnessing the potent therapeutic properties of medicinal plants to support the body's natural detoxification processes.

Dr. Sebi advocates for the use of specific herbs that have been traditionally used for their detoxifying effects and are aligned with his alkaline, plant-based philosophy. These herbs are selected for their ability to stimulate liver function, enhance kidney filtration, promote lymphatic drainage, and support the elimination of toxins from the body.

Among the detoxifying herbs recommended by Dr. Sebi are burdock root, known for its blood-cleansing properties and ability to support liver health. Burdock root aids in the elimination of toxins by enhancing bile production and flow, which helps to detoxify the liver and improve digestion.

Dandelion is another herb favored by Dr. Sebi for its detoxifying effects on the liver and kidneys. Dandelion stimulates bile production, enhances kidney filtration, and acts as a diuretic, promoting the elimination of waste products and toxins from the body through urine.

Milk thistle is renowned for its hepatoprotective properties and its ability to support liver function. This herb contains a compound called silymarin, which helps to regenerate liver cells, reduce inflammation, and protect the liver from damage caused by toxins and free radicals.

Bladderwrack, a type of seaweed, is rich in iodine and other trace minerals that support thyroid function and promote detoxification. Bladderwrack also contains alginate, a compound that binds to heavy metals and facilitates their elimination from the body.

By incorporating these detoxifying herbs into one's daily regimen, individuals can support the body's natural detoxification pathways and promote the cleansing and rejuvenation of vital organs. Dr. Sebi's guide to detoxification empowers readers with the knowledge and tools needed to embark on a journey towards optimal health and vitality through the healing power of medicinal plants.

Alkaline Diet for Detox:

Dr. Sebi's guide to detoxification illuminates the pivotal role of an alkaline diet in promoting detoxification and eliminating acidic waste from the body. Dr. Sebi's holistic approach to detoxification centers around the principle of alkalinity, emphasizing the consumption of alkaline-forming foods to restore the body's natural pH balance and support its inherent detoxification processes.

An alkaline diet primarily consists of plant-based foods that are rich in alkaline minerals such as potassium, magnesium, calcium, and trace minerals. These foods include fruits, vegetables, nuts, seeds, and legumes, which help to alkalize the body and create an environment that is conducive to detoxification.

The alkaline nature of these foods helps to neutralize acidic waste products that accumulate in the body as a result of metabolic processes, dietary choices, and environmental exposures. Acidic waste can lead to inflammation, oxidative stress, and cellular damage if not effectively neutralized and eliminated from the body.

By prioritizing alkaline-forming foods and minimizing acidic foods such as processed foods, animal products, caffeine, and alcohol, individuals can support the body's natural detoxification pathways and promote the elimination of acidic waste products.

In addition to alkaline foods, Dr. Sebi also recommends incorporating alkaline beverages such as herbal teas, fresh fruit juices, and purified water into one's daily regimen. These beverages help to hydrate the body and flush out toxins, further supporting the detoxification process.

By adopting an alkaline diet rich in plant-based foods and alkaline beverages, individuals can create an internal environment that fosters detoxification, cellular repair, and overall well-being. Dr. Sebi's guide to detoxification empowers individuals with the knowledge and tools needed to optimize their health through the transformative power of an alkaline diet.

Juice Fasting and Cleansing:

Dr. Sebi's guide to detoxification introduces readers to the transformative benefits of juice fasting and cleansing protocols as powerful tools to kickstart the detoxification process and rejuvenate the body. Juice fasting involves consuming only fresh, raw fruit and vegetable juices for a designated period, typically ranging from one to several days.

Juice fasting offers numerous benefits for detoxification and overall health. By abstaining from solid foods and nourishing the body with nutrient-dense juices, individuals provide their digestive system with a much-needed rest, allowing it to redirect energy towards cellular repair, detoxification, and renewal. The high concentration of vitamins, minerals, antioxidants, and enzymes found in fresh juices supports the body's natural detoxification pathways and facilitates the elimination of toxins and metabolic waste.

Dr. Sebi's approach to juice fasting emphasizes the importance of selecting organic, locally sourced fruits and vegetables to minimize exposure to pesticides and maximize nutrient content. He recommends a diverse array of juices made from alkaline-forming fruits and vegetables such as green leafy vegetables, celery, cucumber, apples, ginger, and citrus fruits. These juices are rich in chlorophyll, antioxidants, and phytonutrients that promote detoxification, alkalization, and cellular regeneration.

In addition to juice fasting, Dr. Sebi also advocates for periodic cleansing protocols to further support the body's detoxification processes. These protocols may include herbal cleanses, colon hydrotherapy, or sauna therapy, which help to enhance detoxification, stimulate circulation, and promote the elimination of toxins through sweat, urine, and bowel movements.

By incorporating juice fasting and cleansing protocols into one's detoxification regimen, individuals can experience profound transformation on physical, mental, and spiritual levels. These practices serve as catalysts for detoxification, awakening the body's innate healing intelligence and rejuvenating the mind, body, and spirit. Dr. Sebi's guide to detoxification empowers individuals to embark on a journey of self-discovery, renewal, and optimal health through the transformative power of juice fasting and cleansing.

Colon Health and Cleansing:

Dr. Sebi's guide to detoxification highlights the critical role of colon health in the detoxification process and provides insights into supporting a healthy colon through dietary and herbal interventions. The colon, also known as the large intestine, plays a crucial role in eliminating waste products and toxins from the body. However, a congested or sluggish colon can hinder the body's detoxification efforts, leading to toxin buildup, digestive issues, and overall compromised health.

Dr. Sebi emphasizes the importance of maintaining a healthy colon through dietary choices that promote regular bowel movements and optimal digestive function. A diet rich in fiber, obtained from fruits, vegetables, whole grains, and legumes, supports proper colon function by promoting bowel regularity and preventing constipation. Fiber acts as a natural bulking agent, helping to sweep toxins and waste products out of the colon and facilitating their elimination from the body.

In addition to dietary interventions, Dr. Sebi recommends incorporating specific herbal remedies into one's regimen to support colon health and enhance detoxification. These herbs are selected for their ability to stimulate peristalsis, tone the intestinal muscles, and promote healthy bowel movements. Examples of such herbs include cascara sagrada, senna leaf, psyllium husk, and aloe vera.

Colon cleansing protocols, such as herbal enemas or colon hydrotherapy, are also advocated by Dr. Sebi as effective methods for promoting colon health and facilitating detoxification. These protocols help to remove impacted fecal matter, toxins, and parasites from the colon, restoring its natural balance and function. By periodically cleansing the colon, individuals can optimize digestive health, enhance nutrient absorption, and support overall well-being.

Overall, Dr. Sebi's guide to colon health and cleansing emphasizes the importance of maintaining a healthy colon as a cornerstone of the detoxification process. Through dietary modifications, herbal interventions, and colon cleansing protocols, individuals can support their body's natural detoxification pathways, promote colon health, and experience the transformative benefits of optimal digestion and elimination.

Skin Detoxification Techniques:

Dr. Sebi's guide to detoxification delves into his recommendations for skin detoxification, offering insights into various techniques that promote the elimination of toxins through the skin. The skin, the body's largest organ, plays a vital role in detoxification by serving as a barrier that prevents harmful substances from entering the body and facilitating the elimination of toxins through sweat.

Dr. Sebi advocates for holistic approaches to skin detoxification that support the body's natural processes and promote overall well-being. One of the key techniques recommended by Dr. Sebi is herbal baths, which involve soaking in a bath infused with detoxifying herbs such as burdock root, chamomile, lavender, and calendula. These herbs contain compounds that help to draw out impurities, soothe inflammation, and promote relaxation, allowing the body to release toxins through the pores of the skin.

Dry brushing is another technique endorsed by Dr. Sebi for skin detoxification. Dry brushing involves using a natural bristle brush to gently exfoliate the skin and stimulate lymphatic drainage. This practice helps to remove dead skin cells, unclog pores, and promote the elimination of toxins through the lymphatic system. Dry brushing also enhances circulation, which supports overall skin health and vitality.

In addition to herbal baths and dry brushing, Dr. Sebi emphasizes the importance of adopting a natural skincare routine that avoids harsh chemicals and synthetic ingredients. Natural skincare products made from plant-based ingredients nourish and protect the skin without compromising its natural balance. Dr. Sebi recommends using gentle cleansers, moisturizers, and masks that contain herbal extracts, essential oils, and botanical ingredients to support skin detoxification and promote a healthy complexion.

By incorporating skin detoxification techniques such as herbal baths, dry brushing, and natural skincare routines into one's regimen, individuals can support the body's natural detoxification processes and promote radiant, healthy skin from the inside out. Dr. Sebi's guide to skin detoxification empowers individuals to nurture and protect their skin while enhancing overall well-being through holistic self-care practices.

Emotional Detoxification:

Dr. Sebi's guide to detoxification delves into the profound connection between emotional well-being and the detoxification process, offering strategies for releasing emotional toxins stored in the body. Dr. Sebi recognizes that emotional stress, trauma, and unresolved issues can contribute to the accumulation of toxins within the body, leading to imbalances and compromised health. Emotional detoxification involves acknowledging and processing these emotions, allowing them to be released from the body in a healthy and constructive manner. Dr. Sebi advocates for holistic approaches to emotional detoxification, such as mindfulness practices, meditation, journaling, and therapeutic techniques, that promote self-awareness, emotional resilience, and inner peace. By addressing emotional toxins stored in the body, individuals can support their overall detoxification process and experience greater emotional well-being and vitality.

-Detoxification for Weight Loss:

Dr. Sebi explores how detoxification can be a powerful tool for supporting weight loss efforts by improving metabolism, reducing inflammation, and optimizing nutrient absorption. Excess weight and toxins often go hand in hand, as toxins can disrupt metabolic processes, lead to inflammation, and interfere with hormone balance, all of which contribute to weight gain. Detoxification supports weight loss by enhancing the body's ability to metabolize fat, reducing inflammation that can hinder weight loss efforts, and improving nutrient absorption, allowing the body to utilize nutrients more efficiently for energy production and cellular repair. Dr. Sebi advocates for detoxification protocols that emphasize whole, plant-based foods, herbal remedies, and lifestyle modifications that promote detoxification and sustainable weight loss. By adopting a holistic approach to detoxification, individuals can achieve their weight loss goals while simultaneously supporting their overall health and well-being.

Long-Term Detoxification Strategies:

Dr. Sebi provides insights into sustainable detoxification practices that can be incorporated into daily life for long-term health and vitality. While short-term detoxification protocols can provide immediate benefits, long-term detoxification strategies are essential for maintaining optimal health and preventing the accumulation of toxins over time. Dr. Sebi emphasizes the importance of adopting a holistic lifestyle that prioritizes whole, plant-based foods, regular physical activity, stress management techniques, adequate hydration, and restful sleep. These lifestyle practices support the body's natural detoxification processes, promote cellular renewal, and enhance overall vitality. Dr. Sebi also recommends periodic detoxification rituals, such as seasonal cleanses, intermittent fasting, and herbal supplementation, to further support long-term detoxification and rejuvenation. By integrating sustainable detoxification strategies into daily life, individuals can cultivate resilience, vitality, and a deep sense of well-being that lasts a lifetime.

BOOK 23: Dr. Sebi's Holistic Lifestyle

The Mind-Body Connection:

Dr. Sebi's holistic lifestyle teachings emphasize the profound interconnectedness of mental, emotional, and physical health, underscoring how nurturing each aspect contributes to overall well-being. According to Dr. Sebi, the mind-body connection is a fundamental principle of holistic health, recognizing that our thoughts, emotions, and beliefs profoundly influence our physical health and vice versa. Positive mental and emotional states promote harmony within the body, while negative thoughts and emotions can manifest as physical symptoms or illness. Dr. Sebi encourages individuals to cultivate self-awareness, mindfulness, and emotional resilience to foster a positive mind-body connection. Practices such as meditation, visualization, and breathwork are recommended by Dr. Sebi to promote mental clarity, emotional balance, and physical vitality. By nurturing the mind-body connection, individuals can enhance their overall well-being and experience greater harmony, peace, and vitality in their lives.

Nutrition Beyond Food:

Dr. Sebi's holistic approach to nutrition extends beyond the mere selection of foods and emphasizes the importance of how we eat, including mindful eating practices and the art of thorough chewing for optimal digestion. Dr. Sebi recognizes that the manner in which we consume food profoundly impacts our digestion, nutrient absorption, and overall health. Mindful eating involves being fully present and attentive while eating, savoring each bite, and paying attention to hunger and fullness cues. By slowing down and savoring our meals, we can enhance digestion, promote satiety, and prevent overeating. Dr. Sebi also emphasizes the importance of chewing food thoroughly to aid in the breakdown of nutrients and support optimal digestion. Proper chewing allows digestive enzymes in saliva to begin the process of breaking down food, facilitating nutrient absorption and reducing the burden on the digestive system. Dr. Sebi encourages individuals to cultivate mindful eating practices and prioritize chewing food thoroughly as essential components of a holistic approach to nutrition and overall well-being.

The Power of Plant-Based Nutrition:

Dr. Sebi passionately advocates for a plant-based diet rich in alkaline foods as a cornerstone of his holistic lifestyle philosophy, highlighting the transformative effects of this dietary approach on health and vitality. According to Dr. Sebi, the human body thrives on a diet that aligns with its natural alkaline state, which is achieved through the consumption of predominantly plant-based foods. Alkaline foods, such as fresh fruits, vegetables, nuts, seeds, and legumes, support the body's natural detoxification processes, promote cellular regeneration, and create an internal environment that is conducive to health and vitality. By adopting a plant-based diet, individuals can experience a wide range of health benefits, including increased energy levels, improved digestion, enhanced immune function, and reduced risk of chronic disease. Dr. Sebi's holistic approach to nutrition emphasizes the importance of consuming whole, unprocessed foods that are grown organically and free from harmful chemicals and additives. Through the power of plant-based nutrition, individuals can nourish their bodies, minds, and spirits and experience the transformative effects of optimal health and vitality.

Daily Routines for Wellness:

Dr. Sebi encourages individuals to incorporate daily routines and rituals into their lives to promote holistic wellness and balance. These routines serve as anchors that support overall well-being and cultivate a sense of harmony and vitality. Dr. Sebi's recommended daily practices include mindfulness meditation, which helps to reduce stress, promote mental clarity, and enhance emotional resilience. Regular exercise is also emphasized by Dr. Sebi as essential for maintaining physical fitness, supporting cardiovascular health, and improving mood and energy levels. In addition to meditation and exercise, Dr. Sebi advocates for self-care rituals such as journaling, creative expression, and spending time in nature to nourish the soul and replenish the spirit. By incorporating these daily routines into their lives, individuals can create a foundation for holistic wellness that supports them in achieving their highest potential and living life to the fullest.

Creating a Healing Environment:

Dr. Sebi emphasizes the significance of our physical surroundings on our health and well-being, highlighting the importance of creating a healing environment conducive to healing and vitality. Our environment

encompasses not only our immediate surroundings, such as our home and workspace, but also the broader natural world in which we live. Dr. Sebi encourages individuals to cultivate a supportive environment that promotes relaxation, rejuvenation, and optimal health. This may involve decluttering and organizing our living spaces to create a sense of harmony and order, incorporating elements of nature such as plants, natural light, and fresh air to promote a connection with the natural world, and minimizing exposure to toxins and pollutants that can compromise health. Dr. Sebi also emphasizes the importance of emotional and social support in creating a healing environment, fostering positive relationships, and surrounding ourselves with supportive and nurturing individuals who uplift and inspire us. By consciously designing our environment to support our health and well-being, we can create a space that nourishes our body, mind, and spirit and facilitates our journey towards optimal health and vitality.

Connecting with Nature: Dr. Sebi extols the healing power of nature and emphasizes the importance of spending time outdoors, connecting with natural elements, and grounding oneself in the Earth's energy as essential components of his holistic lifestyle. Nature has a profound ability to heal, rejuvenate, and restore balance to the mind, body, and spirit. Dr. Sebi encourages individuals to immerse themselves in nature regularly, whether it be through walks in the park, hiking in the mountains, swimming in the ocean, or simply spending time in a garden or green space. By connecting with natural elements such as trees, plants, water, and sunlight, we can tap into the Earth's energy, absorb healing vibrations, and experience a sense of peace, serenity, and connection with all living things. Dr. Sebi also emphasizes the importance of grounding, or earthing, which involves direct contact with the Earth's surface, such as walking barefoot on grass or soil. Grounding allows us to absorb the Earth's electrons, reduce inflammation, and promote balance within the body. By cultivating a deep connection with nature and incorporating outdoor activities into our daily lives, we can enhance our overall health and well-being and experience the transformative power of nature in our lives.

Cultivating Positive Relationships:

Dr. Sebi recognizes the profound impact of relationships on our health and well-being and emphasizes the importance of cultivating supportive, nourishing connections in alignment with his holistic lifestyle principles. Positive relationships are essential for our emotional, mental, and physical health, providing us with love, support, and a sense of belonging. Dr. Sebi encourages individuals to surround themselves with people who uplift, inspire, and empower them to be their best selves. This may involve fostering deeper connections with family members, friends, and community members who share similar values and aspirations. Dr. Sebi also emphasizes the importance of setting boundaries and prioritizing relationships that nourish and support our growth and well-being while releasing toxic or draining connections that no longer serve us. By cultivating positive relationships based on mutual respect, trust, and understanding, we can create a supportive network of individuals who encourage us to thrive and live life to the fullest in alignment with Dr. Sebi's holistic lifestyle principles.

Stress Management Techniques:

Dr. Sebi recognizes the profound impact of stress on our health and well-being and offers practical strategies for managing stress and cultivating resilience in alignment with his holistic approach to health. Stress is an inevitable part of life, but how we respond to it can significantly influence our physical, mental, and emotional health. Dr. Sebi advocates for holistic stress management techniques that address the root causes of stress and promote balance and harmony in our lives. These techniques may include mindfulness meditation, deep breathing exercises, yoga, tai chi, and qigong, which help to activate the body's relaxation response, reduce cortisol levels, and promote a sense of calm and inner peace. Dr. Sebi also emphasizes the importance of self-care practices such as regular exercise, adequate sleep, healthy nutrition, and spending time in nature to recharge and rejuvenate our body and mind. By incorporating these stress management techniques into our daily routine, we can build resilience, enhance our ability to cope with life's challenges, and cultivate a deep sense of well-being and vitality.

Embracing Spirituality:

Dr. Sebi views spirituality as an integral component of holistic health, recognizing the interconnectedness of the mind, body, and spirit in achieving overall well-being. Spirituality encompasses a deep sense of connection to something greater than oneself, whether it be a higher power, the universe, or the divine essence within. Dr. Sebi encourages individuals to explore their spiritual beliefs and practices as a means of nurturing inner peace, purpose, and fulfillment. This may involve meditation, prayer, mindfulness practices, or engaging in sacred rituals and ceremonies that resonate with one's spiritual path. By cultivating a deeper connection to our innermost selves and the spiritual realm, we can tap into a source of wisdom, guidance, and healing that transcends the physical realm. Spirituality provides a sense of meaning, purpose, and direction in life, helping us navigate challenges, find solace in times of adversity, and cultivate a sense of inner peace and harmony. Dr. Sebi's holistic lifestyle promotes the integration of spirituality into all aspects of daily life, recognizing its profound influence on our health, happiness, and overall well-being.

Living in Alignment with Nature:

Dr. Sebi advocates for living in harmony with the natural rhythms of the Earth and the seasons as a means of promoting balance and vitality in all aspects of life. Nature operates in cycles, with each season bringing its own unique energy, rhythms, and opportunities for growth and renewal. Dr. Sebi encourages individuals to attune themselves to these natural cycles and align their daily activities, habits, and routines with the rhythms of nature. This may involve observing the changing seasons, eating seasonally and locally grown foods, and engaging in activities that reflect the energy of each season, such as outdoor exercise in the spring, swimming in the summer, harvesting and preserving foods in the fall, and practicing introspection and reflection in the winter. By living in harmony with nature, we can optimize our health, enhance our vitality, and experience a deeper connection to the natural world and all living beings. Dr. Sebi's holistic lifestyle emphasizes the importance of respecting and honoring the Earth as a source of nourishment, wisdom, and life force energy, and encourages individuals to cultivate a deep reverence for the interconnected web of life of which we are all a part.

BOOK 24: Dr. Sebi's Herbal First Aid

Introduction to Herbal First Aid:

Dr. Sebi's Herbal First Aid introduces readers to the principles behind herbal first aid and its crucial role in addressing minor health concerns and emergencies. Herbal first aid involves the use of medicinal herbs and natural remedies to treat common injuries, ailments, and accidents that may occur in everyday life. Unlike conventional first aid, which often relies on synthetic medications and treatments, herbal first aid harnesses the healing power of nature to promote natural healing and support the body's innate ability to heal itself. Dr. Sebi emphasizes the importance of empowering individuals with the knowledge and skills to address minor health issues independently using safe, effective, and natural remedies derived from medicinal plants. Herbal first aid is not only practical and cost-effective but also aligns with Dr. Sebi's holistic approach to health, which emphasizes the importance of treating the root causes of illness and supporting the body's natural healing processes.

Essential Herbs for First Aid:

Dr. Sebi's Herbal First Aid highlights essential herbs recommended by Dr. Sebi for addressing common first aid situations, such as cuts, burns, insect bites, and minor infections. These herbs possess potent medicinal properties that help to soothe inflammation, promote tissue repair, and prevent infection, making them invaluable additions to any herbal first aid kit. Some of the essential herbs featured in Dr. Sebi's Herbal First Aid include aloe vera, known for its cooling and soothing properties that aid in treating burns and skin irritations; calendula, prized for its antibacterial and wound-healing properties that accelerate the healing of cuts and abrasions; lavender, renowned for its analgesic and antiseptic properties that alleviate pain and prevent infection in minor wounds; and tea tree oil, celebrated for its antimicrobial and anti-inflammatory properties that combat bacterial and fungal infections and relieve itching and inflammation associated with insect bites and stings.

By familiarizing themselves with these essential herbs and their therapeutic uses, individuals can confidently and effectively address minor health concerns and emergencies using natural remedies derived from medicinal plants, in alignment with Dr. Sebi's holistic approach to health and healing.

Preparation and Application:

Dr. Sebi's Herbal First Aid equips readers with the knowledge and skills to prepare and administer herbal remedies for various first aid situations. Understanding how to properly prepare and apply herbal remedies is essential for maximizing their effectiveness and promoting healing. Dr. Sebi provides detailed instructions on how to create herbal poultices, tablets, tinctures, and salves, which are versatile and convenient forms of herbal preparations for addressing minor health concerns and emergencies. Herbal poultices involve applying a mixture of crushed or powdered herbs directly to the affected area, providing localized relief and promoting healing. Tablets and tinctures are convenient oral forms of herbal remedies that can be easily administered for internal use, allowing for systemic effects and long-lasting relief. Salves, or herbal ointments, are topical preparations that contain herbal extracts infused into a base such as beeswax or coconut oil, providing a soothing and protective barrier over the skin while delivering the healing properties of the herbs. By learning how to prepare and apply herbal remedies in various forms, individuals can effectively address a wide range of first aid situations and promote natural healing in alignment with Dr. Sebi's holistic approach to health and well-being.

Herbal Remedies for Pain Relief:

Dr. Sebi's Herbal First Aid introduces readers to a selection of herbal remedies recommended by Dr. Sebi for natural pain relief. Pain is a common symptom associated with various health conditions and injuries, and herbal remedies offer safe and effective alternatives to conventional pain medications. Dr. Sebi highlights specific herbs known for their analgesic and anti-inflammatory properties, which can help alleviate pain and discomfort associated with headaches, muscle aches, joint pain, and menstrual cramps. Some of the herbs featured in Dr. Sebi's Herbal First Aid for pain relief include feverfew, valued for its ability to reduce the frequency and intensity of headaches and migraines; turmeric, prized for its potent anti-inflammatory properties that relieve pain and inflammation in muscles and joints; white willow bark, renowned for its natural pain-relieving properties similar to aspirin; and cramp bark, traditionally used to ease menstrual cramps and abdominal discomfort. By incorporating these herbal remedies into their first aid toolkit, individuals can effectively manage pain and discomfort naturally, without the risk of side effects associated with conventional pain medications, in alignment with Dr. Sebi's holistic approach to health and healing.

Herbal Remedies for Digestive Issues:

Dr. Sebi's Herbal First Aid delves into herbal remedies for addressing common digestive complaints, offering relief and promoting digestive wellness. Digestive issues such as indigestion, bloating, nausea, and diarrhea can significantly impact daily life and overall well-being. Dr. Sebi advocates for the use of natural herbal remedies to alleviate these symptoms and restore balance to the digestive system. Some of the herbs featured in Dr. Sebi's Herbal First Aid for digestive support include peppermint, valued for its ability to soothe indigestion, relieve gas and bloating, and ease nausea; ginger, renowned for its anti-inflammatory and carminative properties that aid in digestion and alleviate gastrointestinal discomfort; fennel, prized for its digestive benefits, including reducing bloating, relieving gas, and promoting healthy digestion; and chamomile, known for its calming and anti-inflammatory properties that soothe the digestive tract and ease symptoms of indigestion and upset stomach.

By incorporating these herbal remedies into their first aid regimen, individuals can effectively address digestive issues naturally and promote digestive wellness in alignment with Dr. Sebi's holistic approach to health and healing.

Herbal Solutions for Respiratory Support:

Dr. Sebi's Herbal First Aid provides insights into herbs that support respiratory health and offer relief from symptoms of coughs, colds, congestion, and allergies. Respiratory issues such as coughs, congestion, and allergies can be disruptive and uncomfortable, affecting breathing and overall quality of life. Dr. Sebi recommends herbal remedies that help clear congestion, soothe irritated airways, and support respiratory function. Some of the herbs highlighted in Dr. Sebi's Herbal First Aid for respiratory support include eucalyptus, valued for its decongestant and expectorant properties that help clear congestion and promote easy breathing; licorice root, renowned for its soothing and anti-inflammatory effects on the respiratory tract, relieving coughs and reducing throat irritation; mullein, prized for its ability to loosen mucus and ease coughs, making it beneficial for respiratory conditions such as bronchitis and asthma; and nettle, known for its anti-inflammatory properties that help alleviate allergy symptoms and support overall respiratory health. By incorporating these herbal solutions into their first aid kit, individuals can effectively manage respiratory issues and promote respiratory wellness naturally, in alignment with Dr. Sebi's holistic approach to health and healing.

Herbal Support for Stress and Anxiety: Dr. Sebi's Herbal First Aid introduces readers to calming herbs and adaptogens that aid in relieving stress, anxiety, and tension, promoting a sense of calm and emotional well-being. In today's fast-paced world, stress and anxiety have become prevalent issues that can impact mental, emotional, and physical health. Dr. Sebi advocates for the use of natural herbal remedies to help individuals manage stress and anxiety effectively. Calming herbs such as chamomile, passionflower, and lemon balm are known for their soothing properties that help calm the nervous system, reduce anxiety, and promote relaxation. Adaptogens such as ashwagandha, holy basil, and rhodiola rosea help the body adapt to stress, increase resilience, and restore balance to the adrenal glands. By incorporating these herbal remedies into their first aid toolkit, individuals can support their body's natural stress response, improve their ability to cope with stressors, and cultivate a greater sense of calm and emotional well-being in alignment with Dr. Sebi's holistic approach to health and healing.

-Herbal Remedies for Skin Conditions: Dr. Sebi's Herbal First Aid explores herbal recommendations for addressing common skin conditions, offering solutions to promote healthy skin from the inside out. Skin conditions such as rashes, eczema, psoriasis, and acne can be distressing and impact self-confidence and overall well-being. Dr. Sebi advocates for a holistic approach to skin health that addresses underlying imbalances in the body and supports skin healing and rejuvenation. Some of the herbs highlighted in Dr. Sebi's Herbal First Aid for skin conditions include burdock root, valued for its blood-purifying and anti-inflammatory properties that help clear skin impurities and support detoxification; sarsaparilla, renowned for its skin-clearing and detoxifying effects that alleviate skin conditions such as acne and eczema; dandelion, prized for its liver-cleansing and skin-healing properties that improve skin health from the inside out; and calendula, known for its soothing and anti-inflammatory effects that calm irritated skin and promote healing of rashes and eczema. By incorporating these herbal remedies into their first aid regimen, individuals can address skin conditions naturally and promote healthy, radiant skin in alignment with Dr. Sebi's holistic approach to health and healing.

Herbal First Aid Kits:

Dr. Sebi's Herbal First Aid provides guidance on assembling and maintaining herbal first aid kits for home and travel, ensuring individuals have access to natural remedies for unexpected emergencies. A well-stocked herbal first aid kit is an essential resource for addressing minor health concerns and injuries effectively and naturally. Dr. Sebi recommends including a variety of herbs, herbal preparations, and essential oils in the first aid kit, along with basic supplies such as bandages, gauze, and scissors. Herbal remedies for common ailments such as cuts, burns, insect bites, digestive issues, and respiratory complaints should be included, along with instructions for their use. By assembling a herbal first aid kit, individuals can be prepared to handle minor health emergencies confidently and effectively, promoting self-reliance and natural healing in alignment with Dr. Sebi's holistic approach to health and well-being.

Empowerment Through Herbal Knowledge:

Dr. Sebi's Herbal First Aid empowers readers with the knowledge and skills to address minor health concerns naturally and effectively using herbal remedies. By gaining a deeper understanding of herbal first aid techniques and remedies, individuals can take control of their health and well-being and become more self-reliant in managing minor health issues. Dr. Sebi's emphasis on herbal knowledge and empowerment encourages individuals to become proactive in their health care and explore natural alternatives to conventional treatments. Armed with the confidence and expertise gained from Dr. Sebi's herbal first aid techniques, individuals can navigate minor health concerns with ease, knowing they have the tools and resources to support their health naturally. This empowerment fosters a sense of confidence, resilience, and self-reliance, empowering individuals to take charge of their health and well-being in alignment with Dr. Sebi's holistic approach to health and healing.

BOOK 25: Dr. Sebi's Wisdom for Longevity

Understanding the Aging Process: Dr. Sebi's Wisdom for Longevity delves into the intricacies of the aging process, offering insights into the factors that contribute to aging according to Dr. Sebi's perspective. Aging is a natural biological process characterized by gradual changes in cells, tissues, and organs over time. Dr. Sebi highlights key factors that accelerate the aging process, including oxidative stress, inflammation, and cellular degeneration. Oxidative stress occurs when there is an imbalance between free radicals and antioxidants in the body, leading to cellular damage and accelerated aging. Chronic inflammation, triggered by factors such as poor diet, stress, and environmental toxins, also plays a significant role in aging by promoting tissue damage and impairing cellular function. Additionally, cellular degeneration, resulting from genetic factors, lifestyle choices, and environmental exposures, contributes to the decline in organ function and overall health associated with aging. By understanding these underlying mechanisms of aging, individuals can take proactive steps to mitigate their effects and promote healthy aging and longevity in alignment with Dr. Sebi's holistic approach to health and well-being.

Nutritional Strategies for Longevity: Dr. Sebi's Wisdom for Longevity introduces readers to dietary recommendations and lifestyle practices that promote longevity and vitality according to Dr. Sebi's teachings. Nutrition plays a crucial role in supporting health and well-being, and Dr. Sebi advocates for a plant-based diet rich in alkaline foods, antioxidants, and anti-inflammatory herbs to promote longevity. Alkaline foods help maintain the body's pH balance and reduce inflammation, supporting cellular health and longevity. Antioxidants, found abundantly in fruits, vegetables, and herbs, neutralize free radicals and protect cells from oxidative damage, slowing the aging process and promoting overall health. Anti-inflammatory herbs, such as turmeric, ginger, and garlic, help reduce inflammation and support immune function, further enhancing longevity and vitality. By incorporating these nutritional strategies into their diet and lifestyle, individuals can optimize their health, promote longevity, and enjoy a vibrant and fulfilling life in alignment with Dr. Sebi's holistic approach to health and well-being.

The Role of Detoxification:

Dr. Sebi's Wisdom for Longevity sheds light on the crucial role of detoxification in promoting longevity and overall well-being. Detoxification is the process by which the body eliminates accumulated toxins and waste products, restoring balance and supporting optimal organ function. Dr. Sebi emphasizes the importance of detoxification for longevity by reducing oxidative stress, inflammation, and cellular damage associated with toxin exposure. Through methods such as fasting, herbal cleanses, and dietary modifications, individuals can support their body's natural detoxification pathways and enhance their capacity to eliminate harmful substances. By eliminating toxins and reducing oxidative stress, detoxification helps to protect cells and tissues from damage, slow the aging process, and promote longevity. Dr. Sebi's holistic approach to health recognizes the importance of detoxification as a foundational principle for achieving and maintaining vitality and longevity.

Physical Activity and Longevity:

Dr. Sebi's Wisdom for Longevity underscores the significance of regular physical activity in promoting longevity and overall vitality. Physical activity plays a crucial role in maintaining muscle tone, cardiovascular health, and overall physical function as we age. Dr. Sebi advocates for a balanced approach to exercise that incorporates both aerobic and strength training activities to promote cardiovascular fitness, muscle strength, and flexibility. Regular physical activity helps to improve circulation, support immune function, and reduce the risk of chronic diseases such as heart disease, diabetes, and osteoporosis. Additionally, exercise stimulates the release of endorphins, neurotransmitters that promote feelings of well-being and reduce stress and anxiety. By engaging in regular physical activity, individuals can enhance their quality of life, maintain independence, and enjoy greater vitality and longevity as they age. Dr. Sebi's holistic approach to health emphasizes the importance of integrating physical activity into daily life to support overall well-being and longevity.

Mental and Emotional Well-Being:

Dr. Sebi's Wisdom for Longevity delves into the importance of mental and emotional well-being in promoting longevity and overall health. Cultivating positive mental and emotional states is essential for maintaining resilience, reducing stress, and enhancing overall well-being as we age. Dr. Sebi advocates for practices such as mindfulness, gratitude, and stress management to support mental and emotional health. Mindfulness practices, such as meditation and deep breathing exercises, help individuals cultivate present moment awareness, reduce anxiety, and promote a sense of calm and clarity. Gratitude practices encourage individuals to focus on the positive aspects of their lives, fostering feelings of contentment and well-being. Stress management techniques, such as relaxation techniques and positive coping strategies, help individuals effectively navigate life's challenges and reduce the harmful effects of chronic stress on the body and mind. By prioritizing mental and emotional well-being and incorporating these practices into daily life, individuals can promote longevity, resilience, and overall quality of life in alignment with Dr. Sebi's holistic approach to health and well-being.

Connecting with Purpose:

Dr. Sebi's Wisdom for Longevity explores the significance of having a sense of purpose and meaning in life for promoting longevity and overall well-being. Having a clear sense of purpose and meaning provides individuals with a sense of direction, motivation, and fulfillment that contributes to overall well-being and longevity. Dr. Sebi encourages individuals to explore their passions, values, and goals to discover their unique purpose in life. Connecting with purpose involves aligning one's actions and choices with their core values and aspirations, leading to a sense of fulfillment and satisfaction. Research has shown that having a sense of purpose is associated with better physical and mental health outcomes, reduced risk of chronic diseases, and increased longevity. By nurturing a sense of purpose and meaning in life, individuals can enhance their quality of life, promote resilience, and enjoy greater vitality and longevity. Dr. Sebi's holistic approach to health emphasizes the importance of connecting with purpose as a fundamental aspect of promoting overall well-being and longevity.

Social Connections and Community:

Dr. Sebi's Wisdom for Longevity explores the vital role of social connections and community involvement in promoting longevity and overall well-being. Strong social connections and a sense of belonging are essential for maintaining emotional health, reducing stress, and enhancing resilience as we age. Dr. Sebi emphasizes the importance of nurturing meaningful relationships with family, friends, and community members to support longevity. Engaging in social activities, participating in group events, and volunteering in the community are all ways to foster social connections and strengthen social support networks. Research has shown that individuals with strong social connections tend to live longer, healthier lives compared to those who are socially isolated. By prioritizing social connections and community involvement, individuals can enhance their quality of life, promote longevity, and enjoy a greater sense of belonging and fulfillment in alignment with Dr. Sebi's holistic approach to health and well-being.

Environmental Factors:

Dr. Sebi's Wisdom for Longevity delves into the impact of environmental factors on longevity and overall health. Environmental factors such as air and water quality, exposure to toxins, and access to green spaces can significantly influence health outcomes and life expectancy. Dr. Sebi highlights the importance of minimizing exposure to environmental toxins and pollutants to promote longevity and well-being. This includes reducing exposure to air pollution, drinking clean and filtered water, and avoiding exposure to harmful chemicals and pesticides. Additionally, Dr. Sebi encourages individuals to seek out green spaces and natural environments, as spending time in nature has been shown to reduce stress, improve mood, and promote overall health. By being mindful of environmental factors and taking steps to mitigate their effects, individuals can optimize their living environment and support longevity and vitality in alignment with Dr. Sebi's holistic approach to health and well-being.

Spiritual Practices

Dr. Sebi's Wisdom for Longevity delves into the profound role of spirituality in promoting longevity and overall well-being. Spirituality encompasses a wide range of beliefs and practices that connect individuals with a higher power, inner wisdom, and the deeper meaning of life. Dr. Sebi advocates for spiritual practices such as meditation, prayer, and connecting with higher consciousness as powerful tools for promoting longevity and vitality. Meditation allows individuals to quiet the mind, cultivate inner peace, and access deeper levels of awareness and insight. Prayer provides a channel for expressing gratitude, seeking guidance, and fostering a sense of connection with the divine. Connecting with higher consciousness involves transcending the ego and aligning with the universal intelligence that permeates all of existence. By incorporating spiritual practices into daily life, individuals can nurture their spiritual well-being, cultivate inner peace, and enhance their sense of purpose and fulfillment. Dr. Sebi's holistic approach to health recognizes the profound connection between spirituality and longevity, encouraging individuals to explore and embrace their spiritual nature as a pathway to optimal health and well-being.

Integrating Dr. Sebi's Wisdom:

Dr. Sebi's Wisdom for Longevity provides practical insights into how to integrate Dr. Sebi's teachings for longevity into daily life. Integrating Dr. Sebi's wisdom involves incorporating his dietary recommendations, lifestyle practices, and holistic principles into your daily routine to foster health, vitality, and a sense of purpose as you age. This may include adopting a plant-based diet rich in alkaline foods, incorporating regular physical activity, prioritizing mental and emotional well-being, nurturing social connections, and engaging in spiritual practices. By aligning with Dr. Sebi's holistic approach to health and wellness, individuals can optimize their physical, mental, emotional, and spiritual well-being, promoting longevity and vitality as they age. Integrating Dr. Sebi's wisdom into daily life is an ongoing journey of self-discovery, self-care, and personal growth, guided by the principles of balance, harmony, and alignment with nature. Through conscious choices and mindful living, individuals can cultivate health, vitality, and a profound sense of well-being that enriches every aspect of life.

"Here you will find your bonuses".

Conclusion

Whether you have a history of chronic inflammation, following an anti-inflammatory meal is a smart way to eat. Anti-inflammatory eating is a lifestyle, adds Scanniello, and this will improve your well-being, health, and general quality of life in the end. Anyone can take advantage of a food plan like this, and I've found it particularly useful in individuals suffering from chronic inflammation and health issues."

You'll probably begin to feel significantly better when you eat this way. Scanniello believes that "people may have decreased bloating, gastrointestinal pain, and aches." You could also notice a shift in your emotions due to making dietary changes.

Don't anticipate fast results from a health problem; it may take almost twelve weeks to see the long-term or short-term outcomes, depending on the situation.

There are no serious drawbacks as long as you stick to the anti-inflammatory diet and understand which items to consume and which ones to avoid.

You may have a time of transition if your present diet consists of processed foods and dairy. As a result, you'll need to spend more effort and time preparing your meals, and you won't be able to stop for processed food while on this strategy.

A diet based on an anti-inflammatory approach entail eating many foods proven to reduce inflammation and limiting your consumption of foods that do the reverse. However, one of the nicest aspects of the diet is a wide variety of meals to select from and plenty of wiggle space.

The Mediterranean diet is a good option if you're looking for more organization in your eating habits. Because both diets stress eating fruits, veggies, & whole grains, there is a massive overlap. Preventing disease progression, reducing medication use and reducing joint injury are possible outcomes of an anti-inflammation and alkaline diet.

Made in the USA
Columbia, SC
23 June 2024

37415898R00204